MEDITERRANEAN DIET PLAN:

The First Complete Guide

Mediterranean Diet, Cookbook and Healthy Recipes for Burn Fat, Plant, Reset your Metabolism and Weight Loss,

4-Week Mediterranean diet Plan,

Mindset Paradox for Success

Table of Contents

Introduction

Congratulations on downloading the *MEDITERRANEAN DIET PLAN: The First Complete Guide Mediterranean Diet, Cookbook And Recipes, Plan, Guide With Exercise For Weight Loss, 4-Week Mediterranean Diet Plan, Mindset Paradox For Success.* Thank you for doing so. I am so excited that you have chosen to take a new path using the Mediterranean way of eating. Before we proceed, here's a bit of history.

Ancel Keys, a scientist, and his colleagues including Paul Dudley which later became President Eisenhower's cardiac physician conducted a *Seven Countries Study* in the years following World War II. The study compared individuals in the United States to those living in Crete - a Mediterranean island. Keys examined the plan testing people of all ages using the Mediterranean Diet.

The study examined 13,000 middle-aged men in Finland, the United States, the Netherlands, Yugoslavia, Greece, Italy, and Japan. It became evident the fruits, vegetables, grains, beans, and fish were the healthiest meals possible - even after the impoverishment of WWII. All of these discoveries were just the starting point.

Many benefits will be discussed including how you can lose and maintain a healthy weight in a sustainable way. Each chapter will carry you through different aspects of the plan and how you can go about changing your eating patterns with the Mediterranean diet.

You will also discover while on the Mediterranean diet plan, you will have more energy, and with that energy, you can become more active. Motivation will be the leader as you head toward your new lifestyle making essential changes along the path to success. Now it's time to learn how to use the techniques of the Mediterranean Diet Plan.

After you have the basics, you will enjoy a 28-day menu plan with all of the recipes included. Let's Get Started!

Chapter 1: Why the Mediterranean Diet?

The Mediterranean way of eating is typically rich in healthy plant foods and lower in animal foods. It places more of a focus on fish and seafood. It is predominantly beneficial because, at the end of the day, you won't be hungry!

The Mediterranean diet emphasizes that you get plenty of exercises, and primarily consume foods such as fruits, vegetables, legumes and nuts, and whole grains. You should consider replacing butter with healthier fats including canola or olive oil. Instead of salt, use spices and different herbs. Stick by the Mediterranean pyramid of foods and you won't go wrong!

Enjoy meals with family and friends using your new-found recipes and methods. Enjoy poultry and fish at least twice a week and have an occasional glass of red wine.

Health Benefits

The Mediterranean Plan is built upon healthy fats as well as plant-based foods.
Since the plan does not eliminate entire food groups, it is believed you should not have any problems complying with it in the long term.

You will have a lowered risk of strokes and heart disease. Patients who use the plan have had lowered level of oxidized low-density lipoprotein or LDL cholesterol. This is the bad cholesterol that can build up in your arteries.

The Mediterranean diet is rich in alpha-linolenic acid which is found in extra-virgin olive oil. The Warwick Medical School involved participants in a study who consumed more EVOO versus sunflower oil. The olive oil totals were much higher for decreased blood pressure. Lowered hypertension is another benefit achieved by consuming olive oil because it helps keep the arteries clear and dilated. It makes the nitric oxide more bioavailable. The healthy fats also make you less likely to struggle to maintain cholesterol levels.

Strokes can be caused by bleeding in the brain or a blocked blood vessel. You may notice numbness, weakness, headaches, confusion, vision problems dizziness, or slurred speech. The diet helps with these issues.

Your vision will improve. You might be able to stave off - or even prevent the risk of macular degeneration which is the major cause for adults over 54 losing their eyesight. The condition affects over ten million Americans and can destroy the area of your retina which is responsible for clear vision. The vegetables and fish with the omega-3 fatty acids are the providers to lower or reduce the risk entirely. Also, you will have less chance of having cataracts with the consumption of green leafy veggies which have lutein.

You will drop the pounds using healthier practices. Your search is over if you are seeking a plan that is worthwhile. The Med Plan, as it is sometimes called, has been proven to work for weight loss easily and naturally with its many nutrient-dense foods. The focus is placed on healthy fats to keep the carbs moderately low and improve high-quality proteins. The healthy fats, protein, and fiber keep you much more satisfied than candy, chips, or cookies. The veggies make up the bulk of the meal by filling your stomach, so you don't feel hungry an hour after your meal, and you won't receive a spike your blood sugar.

You will experience improved agility. Studies have shown up to 70% of the seniors who are at risk of developing frailty or other muscle weaknesses have reduced the risks factors using the plan.

You will enjoy eating natural foods. The Mediterranean diet is low in sugar and processed foods. You can certainly appreciate a diet or a way of life that is close to nature, especially if you can locate some locally produced organic sources. People in the Mediterranean enjoy the same types of delicious desserts and many are made using natural sweeteners such as honey.

Improved asthma symptoms are evident from those using the plan. Numerous studies have revealed the antioxidant diet helped children who followed the plan emphasizing the intake of plant-based foods and lower intake of red meats.

Risk factors for Alzheimer's are reduced. Research has deemed a 40% reduction occurs for those who use the diet plan, and the risk factors associated with Alzheimer's. Dementia may progress in the later stages of Alzheimer's which can be treated with medication and aided by the Mediterranean plan. You should also consider some additional exercise to slow the process.

Reduction in Parkinson's risk factors has been observed. The risk of the disease is cut in half because the high levels of antioxidants in the diet prevent oxidative stress, which is the cell-damaging process. Parkinson's disease affects the cells in your brain which produce dopamine. You may have some issues with gait and speech patterns, tremors, and muscle rigidity issues. The Mediterranean diet can help safeguard you from Alzheimer's which are triggered by thinking, judgment, and memory losses.

The Mediterranean Plan has helped those with diabetes. The Mediterranean Diet controls excessive insulin which is a hormone that controls your blood sugar levels and can cause you to gain weight and keep it on, no matter what you do to try to lose it. The well-balanced diet which is low in sugar and contains healthy fatty acids can create a balance so your body can burn off the fat and give you more energy at the same time.

The diet is considered lower in saturated fat, but higher in fat than the American standard diet plans, according to the *American Heart Association*. The combination is usually 20-30% quality protein foods, 30-40% healthy fats, and 40% complex carbs. This creates the balance to keep your hunger under control and the weight gain down which is an excellent way to keep insulin levels normalized.

As a result, with the energy levels up, so should your mood. Sugar is usually consumed through dessert, fruit, or wine. The balance also prevents the 'highs and lows' which is the mood- altering factor. Most individuals on the plan will eat a balanced breakfast within one or two hours from the time the day starts, which is the time of day the lowest levels of blood sugar are present in the healthy fats and fibers, along with three meals each day to maintain the balance.

The Delicious Path to Weight Loss

You can plan healthy choices for breakfast, lunch, and dinner, but what about your snacking habits? You should choose a healthy snack which would be around the 150-200 calorie marker. Choose a grapefruit, apple, or pear. Add a pinch (⅛ of a teaspoon) of sea salt for a change. This treat will help fend off the hunger cravings. You want it to contain some whole-grain sources, some carbs, and protein to promote satiety.

The path to weight loss is the best way to lose weight using healthy food choices. These are just a few examples of some of the foods you can enjoy when you just do not have the time for a meal:

Nut Butter & Fruit Slices: Pears and apples are a hit when you prepare your favorite nut butter. Cashew butter and almond butter are two healthy choices that contain heart-healthy fats. By roasting and blending the raw almonds, you are ensured to receive all of the rich fiber, protein, and fats that your body needs to remain active.

Dates & Figs: These are some products which grow well in the Mediterranean climate. They are also a sweet treat when you are too busy to prepare a snack.

Tuna Salad & Crackers: It is time to move away from the traditional tuna salad. Substitute oil-packed tuna with a splash of red vinegar wine, scallions, and a squeeze of mustard. Add some whole wheat crackers for a mid-morning treat.

Greek Yogurt & Fruit: Enjoy a protein-rich snack of some Greek yogurt. Garnish the yogurt with some sunflower seeds, a handful of berries, and a drizzle of honey for a tasty mid-afternoon snack.

Sun-Dried Tomato & Goat Cheese Spread: The rich flavor of the sun-dried tomatoes are only the beginning since it is full of calcium, iron, vitamin C, vitamin A, and lycopene. It also provides a heart-healthy boost since it is often packed in olive oil. Smear a layer of goat cheese on whole wheat crackers and top it off with some sun-dried tomatoes for a quick snack. Add a snip of basil on top of each cracker for a few additional vitamins and minerals.

Kalamata Olives: When you are in a rush, nothing says it all like a handful of healthy olives. They are rich in many antioxidants including oleic acid, tyrosol, and hydroxytyrosol. Mix them up with a small amount of feta cheese for an additional boost.

Pita & Hummus: You can have some sesame paste (tahini) and chickpeas in the form of hummus. Consider making some at home, but you can also purchase it ready-made. Make sure you read the label and choose one with a limited amount of preservatives. You can choose a whole-wheat piece of pita bread with a hummus spread for a delicious snack.

Chapter 2: Mindset for Your Diet Success

Research has proven time and again that you have to get in the right mindset to drop the unwanted pounds. Shifting your mindset is about how to lose weight from the outside without realizing the intention. Don't expect quick fixes. All it takes is willpower and setting realistic goals to be successful during your journey through the Mediterranean diet weight loss plan.

If you are choosing to drop the pounds and keep them off, you will discover the Mediterranean style is the cure you have been seeking. You have to get motivated to get any plan to work for you. The first step was taken since you purchased this informative guide.

Jot down your goals and the reasons you need to change your eating patterns. As you proceed with your weight loss, keep your motivation in check by referring to those reasons. It will give you a needed boost.

Surround yourself with people that are positive; you will develop emotionally healthy realistic goals. Dropping the pounds will be the result, but first, you need to set goals. You need to make the goals small with sustainable things that you have full control over to be successful. You can make simple goals such as how many servings of fruits you will eat in one day or how many hours of sleep you will have that night.

It is essential for you to recharge and take the evening hours to relax and improve your sleep hygiene. Try to leave work – at work. Deal with the issues when you return. If you are going through a tough time or working long hours, you tend to forget items you may 'munch' on as you are working. Make it a point to write down everything you eat.

Working long hours can be beneficial for knocking off those pounds, but it can also cause you to be restless and can lead to post-workout insomnia if you have worked out or done other strenuous physical activities on your evenings off.
No matter what the case, slow down for at least an hour or more before attempting to retire for the evening.

If you have dieted before, you already know you will reach spans of time where your weight loss will level out. That's merely a segment of weight loss that can't be moderated. All you need to do is remain consistent. The weight loss will return. It is much better to expect problems or roadblocks than it is to believe that the new dieting methods will be smooth sailing.

Set a timeline with realistic goals. Choosing to lose weight is a fantastic move, but you need to be realistic. You might find it helpful to use baby steps to achieve the desired goal. For example, set a goal to lose six pounds in the next five to six weeks when you begin your new Mediterranean diet plan. For most people, healthy benefits are received if you start the plan by losing five to ten percent of your starting weight. It may not be your ideal medically suggested weight, but it is going to lead you toward a healthier weight. Take baby steps.

Consider what you want to change about the way you feel concerning your weight issues. If you notice you are craving sweets, your plan should include a way to reduce your intake down to two times weekly. Provide you and your family with healthier, filling choices such as fruit. However, don't go cold turkey because the plan won't work. Search for a recipe that allows you to taste the sweetness without the additional calories.

After you have adjusted your body to the Mediterranean way of eating, be willing to change your goals as you make progress. By starting small, you leave the door open so you can make more significant challenges as you proceed through the plan.

Make Healthier Food Choices: Make Substitutions:

- **Breadcrumbs**: You can still enjoy your crunchiness by replacing regular breadcrumbs with crushed pork rinds. The good news is that the pork rinds have zero carbs. Next time, enjoy healthier fats.

- **Pasta**: Replace pasta using zucchini. Use a spiralizer and make long ribbons to cover your plate. It is excellent for many dishes served this way.
  For example, you can also prepare spaghetti squash for regular spaghetti.

- **Tortillas**: Get ready to say no to this one which weighs in at approximately 98 grams for just 1 serving. Instead, enjoy a lettuce leaf at about 1 gram per serving. You will still have a healthy crunch to enjoy!

Portion Control

You need to be aware of the foods you are consuming. This takes good management skills. It is important to set guidelines while on the Mediterranean diet plan. You need to gauge each portion of the food that you're eating to ensure you're getting the correct calorie intake daily. The following lists are just a few examples of how you would portion their foods during your dieting journey:

- *Vegetables*: One cup of raw leafy veggies or one-half cup of all others
- *Fruit*: One orange, one apple, one banana, 30 grams: 1.1 ounces of grapes: 7.1 ounces of watermelon or other melons
- *Legumes*: 100 grams (One cup) of dry cooked beans

- *Grains*: 50 to 60 grams (.5 cup) of cooked pasta or rice: One slice of bread is 25 grams (almost an ounce)
- *Dairy*: One cup of yogurt or one cup of milk, 30 grams, or about 1.1 ounces of cheese or 1 egg.
- *Meat*: 60 grams (2.1 ounces) of fish or lean meat
- *Potatoes*: 100 grams (3.5 ounces)
- *Nuts*: 30 grams (1.1 ounces) Sprinkled on foods for flavor or as a snack

With the right combination of foods, you can set and keep your goals.

Imagine Your Future:

I always try to plan for the future since no one is promised tomorrow. The Mediterranean diet will meet your needs because it is a very sustainable diet plan.

Think about it, this book of guidelines will get you off to the right start with your prepared meal plan. All you have to do is take away the foods you don't like and replace them with Mediterranean diet foods that work. Just so you know how well the plan works, take a snapshot now and save it to your phone. After you have a month or so on the plan, take another snapshot and compare the two.

Consider using free apps to help you track your weight loss. You'll want to keep track of what you eat every day. Research has shown individuals who keep records of their food activity will more than likely be successful with weight loss. You will always be able to move forward when you discover any weaknesses that exist in your dieting success.

- MyFitnessPal has been chosen as one of the best apps available to track your macros. It's free to download, but you can also choose to update to a premium plan for higher rates.

- My Food Diary will provide you with the nutritional facts to ensure you have the correct carbohydrate, protein, and fats in your diet plan.

Prepare A Food Journal: If you cheat or go off of your scheduled meal plan, you should still add the additional calories into your daily log. It will be a reminder of your indulgence, but it will help keep you in line. All you need to do is update your journal regularly, and remain totally honest in the journal and write down all items.

By having a journal, you can document your food items from a different perspective on each day. Make comments over which foods you prepared, and whether you liked or disliked them.

You can also include your objectives of the plan; mention how you're doing on the diet, document your thoughts and feelings as well as your experience with others and yourself as you proceed through each week of the menu plan. Use patience and your time, and you'll appreciate the success you will be provided in the end.

Understand Your Cravings: If you have stood by your guideline and followed the plan, you should see a remarkable improvement. If not, don't give up; instead, just make adjustments and keep dieting.

Salty Foods: Your body is craving silicon. Have a few nuts and seeds; just be sure to count them into your daily counts.

Fatty or Oily Foods: The levels of calcium and chloride need repair with some spinach, broccoli, cheese, or fish.

Sugary Foods: Several things can trigger the desire for sugar, but typically phosphorous, and tryptophan are the culprits. Have some chicken, beef, lamb, liver, cheese, cauliflower, or broccoli.

Chocolate: The carbon, magnesium, and chromium levels are requesting a portion of spinach, nuts, and seeds, or some broccoli and cheese.

Chapter 3: Basic Principles

Learn How to Understand Nutrition Labels

Look for Short Ingredient List: The bulk of the food is listed in order according to weight and are usually the first ingredients. If you don't recognize an ingredient, place it back on the shelf! Consider using products that have no more than 5 ingredients. The longer ingredients probably are the result of unnecessary extras including artificial preservatives.

Check Serving Sizes: Packages often time contain more than a single serving. Visualize how many calories and the amount of sugar is in a single container. Thus, you need to check the serving size first.

Discover Calorie Counts: It is essential to check the labels calorie count since they are very important during your process using the Mediterranean diet plan.

Avoid Fats: It's important to remove foods from your diet plan that contain any fully hydrogenated or partially hydrogenated oils.

Check the Percent of Daily Value: The daily value will tell you how many nutrients are in each serving of a packaged item.

Get More Of These Nutrients: Look for calcium, iron, fiber, vitamin A, and vitamin C.

The Label Explained

1. Serving Information At the Top: This provides the size of one serving and per container.
2. Check the total calories per serving and container.
3. Limit certain nutrients from your diet.
4. Provide yourself with plenty of beneficial nutrients
5. Understand the % of daily value section.

Avoid These Foods

- **Added Sugar:** Ice cream, candy, regular soda, plus many others.

- **Refined Oils**: Canola oil, cottonseed oil, soybean oil, etc.

- **Trans fats**: Found in various processed foods such as margarine, added sugar, ice cream, candies, table sugar, soda, and others. Added sugars, sugar-sweetened beverages, refined grains, processed meats, and other highly processed foods.

- **Processed Meat Products**: Hot dogs, processed sausages, bacon

- **Refined Grains**: Pasta made with refined wheat, white bread

Note If You Are Pregnant: You should avoid some of the oily fish such as swordfish, shark, and tuna because some may contain low levels of toxic heavy metals.

What to Eat Rarely:

- **Red meats** (Limit to once each week)

Foods You Can Eat

Seafood and Fish: Mussels, clams, crab, prawns, oysters, shrimp, tuna, mackerel, salmon, trout, sardines, anchovies, and more

Poultry: Turkey, duck, chicken, and more

Eggs: Duck, quail, and chicken eggs

Dairy Products: Contain calcium, B12, and Vitamin A: Greek yogurt, regular yogurt, cheese, plus others

Tubers: Yams, turnips, potatoes, sweet potatoes, etc.

Vegetables: Another excellent choice for fiber, and antioxidants: Cucumbers, carrots, Brussels sprouts, tomatoes, onions, broccoli, cauliflower, spinach, kale, eggplant, artichokes, fennel, etc.

Seeds and Nuts: Provide minerals, vitamins, fiber, and protein: Macadamia nuts, cashews, pumpkin seeds, sunflower seeds, hazelnuts, chestnuts, Brazil nuts, walnuts, almonds, pumpkin seeds, sesame, poppy, and more

Fruits: Excellent choices for vitamin C, antioxidants, and fiber: Peaches, bananas, apples, figs, dates, pears, oranges, strawberries, melons, grapes, etc.

Spices and Herbs: Cinnamon, garlic, pepper, nutmeg, rosemary, sage, mint, basil, parsley, etc.

Whole Grains: Whole grain bread and pasta, buckwheat, whole wheat, barley, corn, whole oats, rye, quinoa, bulgur, couscous

Legumes: Provide vitamins, fiber, carbohydrates, and protein: Chickpeas, pulses, beans, lentils, peanuts, peas

Healthy Fats: Avocado oil, avocados, and olives are excellent fats. The monounsaturated fat which is found in olive oil is a fat that can help reduce the 'bad' cholesterol. The oil has become the traditional fat worldwide with some of the healthiest populations. A great deal of research has been provided showing the oil is a huge plus towards the risk of heart disease because of the antioxidants and fatty acids.

You will still need to pay close attention when purchasing olive oil because it may have been extracted from the olives using chemicals or possibly diluted with other cheaper oils, such as canola and soybean. You need to be aware of refined or light olive or regular oils. The Mediterranean diet plan calls for the use of extra-virgin olive oil because it has been standardized for purity using natural methods providing the sensory qualities of its excellent taste and smell. The oil is high in phenolic antioxidants which makes—real—olive oil beneficial.

Beverage Options: Maintaining a healthy body requires plenty of water, and the Mediterranean diet plan is not any different. Tea and coffee are allowed, but you should avoid fruit juices or sugar-sweetened beverages that contain large amounts of sugar.

White Meats: White meats are high in minerals, protein, and vitamins but you should remove any visible fat and the skin.

Red Meats: You are allowed red meats including lamb, pork, and beef in small quantities. They are rich in minerals, vitamins, and protein—especially iron. Use caution because they do contain more fat—specifically saturated fat—compared to the fat content found in poultry. Don't leave it out entirely; save it for a special dinner or with a stew or casserole.

Potatoes: You have noticed that potatoes are listed in the tubers group because they are a healthy choice, but it will greatly depend on how they are prepared. You receive potassium, Vitamin B, Vitamin C, and some of your daily fiber nutrients. You must consider that they do contain large amounts of starch which can be quickly converted to glucose which can be harmful and place you at some risk of type 2 diabetes. Use simpler methods of cooking them including baking, boiling, and mashing them without butter.

Desserts and Sweets: Biscuits, cakes, and sweets should be consumed in small quantities, as a special treat. Not only is the sugar a temptation for type 2 diabetes; it can also promote tooth decay. Many times, they may also contain higher levels of saturated fats. You can receive some nutritional value, but as a general rule—stick to small portions.

What to Eat in Moderation: Eggs, poultry, milk, butter, yogurt, and cheese

Improve the Flavor of Foods

The use of her herbs and spices provide additional flavor and aroma to your foods while on the diet plan. It will also help reduce the need for salt or fat while you're preparing your meals. Spices and herbs which adhere to the standards of a traditional Mediterranean Diet include chiles, lavender, tarragon, savory, sumac, and zaatar.

These are a few more ways you can benefit from spices and herbs:

Anise Benefits: You can improve digestion as well as help reduce nausea and alleviate cramps. Prepare some anise tea after a meal to help treat indigestion and bloating gas as well as constipation.

Bay Leaf Benefits: Bay leaves contain magnesium, calcium, potassium, and Vitamins A & C. You are promoting your general health and it is also proven to be useful in the treatment of migraines.

Basil Benefits: You can receive aid in digestion, help with gastric diseases, and help reduce flatulence. You can also protect your heart health, help reduce stress and anxiety, and help manage your diabetes. The next time you have dandruff issues, try rubbing them in your scalp after shampooing. The chemicals help eliminate dandruff and dry skin.

Black Pepper Benefits: Pepper promotes nutrient absorption in the tissues all over your body, speeds up your metabolism, and improves digestion. The main ingredient of pepper is a pipeline which gives it the pungent taste. It can boost fat metabolism by as much as 8% for up to several hours after it's ingested. As you will see, it is used throughout your healthy Mediterranean recipes.

Cayenne Pepper Benefits: The secret ingredient in cayenne is the capsaicin which is a natural compound that gives the peppers the fiery heat. This provides a short increase in your metabolism. The peppers are also rich in vitamins, effective as an appetite controller, smoothes out digestion issues, and benefits your heart health.

Sweet & Spicy Cloves Benefits: Add cloves to hot tea for a spicy flavor. The antiseptic and germicidal ingredients in cloves will help with many types of pain including the relief of arthritis pain, gum and tooth pain, aids in digestive problems, and helps to fight infections. Use the oil of clove as an antiseptic to kill bacteria in fungal infections, itchy rashes, bruises, or burns. Just the smell of cloves can help encourage mental creativity.

Ground Chia Seeds Benefits: The seeds can absorb up to 11 times its weight in liquid. Be sure to add plenty of water and soak them for at least 5 minutes before using in your recipes. Otherwise, you will have some uncomfortable digestion after eating them. Be sure to remain hydrated.

Cumin Benefits: The flavor of cumin and has been described as spicy, earthy, nutty, and warm. It's been a long used as traditional medicine. It can help promote digestion and reduce foodborne infections. It is also beneficial for promoting weight loss and improving cholesterol and blood sugar control.

Fennel Benefits: You can receive potassium, sodium, vitamin A, calcium, vitamin C, iron, vitamin B6, and magnesium from fennel. Your bone health will show improvement with the phosphate and calcium which are excellent for your bone structure. Iron and zinc or crucial for the production of collagen. Your heart health is also protected with vitamin C, folate, potassium, and fiber provided in fennel.

Garlic Benefits: Garlic leads the charge on lowering your blood sugar and assisting you in weight loss. It helps control your appetite.

Ginger Benefits: Ginger is an effective diuretic which increases urine elimination. It is also known for his cholesterol-fighting properties, as a metabolism and mobility booster. Ginger also helps fight bloating issues.

Marjoram Benefits: This is used in the diet to promote healthy digestion, assist in the management of type 2 diabetes, helps to rectify hormonal imbalances, and also helps promote restful sleep and a sound mind.

Mint Benefits: Mint can be used for the treatment of nasal congestion, nausea, dizziness, and headaches. It helps to improve blood circulation, improves dental health, and helps colic in infants. Mint helps to prevent dandruff and pesky head lice.

Oregano Benefits: Oregano is very easily added to your diet and is rich in antioxidants and may also help fight bacteria. Oregano is also good for the treatment of the common cold since it helps in reducing infections, helps kill off intestinal parasites, and it's also beneficial in treating menstrual cramps. One huge plus is that it also supports the body with nutrients to help support weight loss and improve digestion.

Parsley Benefits: You can help your skin, prostate, and digestive tract by making use of its high levels of a flavonoid called apigenin. It contains a powerful antioxidant and inflammatory power as well as providing remarkable anti-cancer properties.

Rosemary Benefits: The spice is known to increase hair growth, may help relieve pain, eases stress, and also helps reduce joint inflammation.

Sage Benefits: The leaves of the sage plant are also used to make medicine. It is an excellent source to improve your digestive issues including diarrhea, stomach pain or gastritis, heartburn, and gas or flatulence. It is also beneficial for those who suffer from depression, Alzheimer's disease, memory loss, and so much more.

Tarragon Benefits: The tarragon spice is an excellent choice for maintaining your blood sugar levels, keeping your heart healthy, reduction of inflammation symptoms, improvement of digestive functions, improves central nervous system conditions, and supports healthier eyes.

Thyme Benefits: Thyme is another spice which has been used throughout history for protection from 'Black Death' as well as for embalming. (Not a pretty thought for dinner but interesting nonetheless.) It is also believed to have insecticidal and antibacterial properties. You can use it as an essential oil, as a dried herb or fresh.

As you will notice, the recipes included in your new menu plan have an extensive listing of spices. Not only do they improve your foods, but also they improve your health at the same time!

Keep to the Diet

No more worrying, you are good to 'go' on the Mediterranean diet - even when you're out. Most restaurants are a reasonable choice for you while you are participating in this diet plan. Ask the waiter or waitress to cook your food using extra-virgin olive oil (EVOO) instead of butter. Choose to have a house salad and extra veggies. Have some seafood or other types of fish for the main entrcc. Eat whole-grain bread.

One huge advantage of the Mediterranean diet is that you can be flexible. These are a few additional tips for dining out beginning with the appetizers, entrees, beverages, and lastly desserts. So, let's get started.

Have a healthy snack before you leave home: One of the

easiest ways to remain on your Mediterranean diet while dining out is to take the edge off of your hunger. Enjoy a high-protein and low-calorie snack such as yogurt to help you feel full. It will help you from overeating.

Enjoy a huge glass of ice water before and during your meal. Eliminate the sugary sweet drinks. Water cannot be stressed enough while you are attempting to drop the pounds since it helps keep you hydrated and steers the hunger away.

Suggestions for the Appetizers: Remove the temptation and ask the waiter/waitress not to bring a bread-and-butter basket to the table. If you are hungry, you may be tempted to eat more than you should. Avoid fried appetizers. Stick with some steamed fish or shellfish, mixed salads, broth-based soups, or grilled veggies. Share your appetizer, so you will have a smaller portion.

Suggestions for the Entree Course: Choose from lean pork (center-cut or tenderloin), fish, poultry, or vegetarian choices. If you are bound for red meat—choose the leaner cuts such as flank, sirloin, filet mignon, or a tenderloin. You might also want to consider the beef will have a higher calorie and higher fat count. Ask for substitutes for mashed potatoes, macaroni salad, potato salad, coleslaw, or French fries. Instead, choose a side salad, steamed rice, baked potato, or steamed veggies.

Use caution with sauces. Ask if it is oil based, or if cream or butter in the sauce. Avoid sauces with cream, cheese, oil, or butter. Request that the sauces be served in a separate container, so you can add what is allowed. Use your fork to dip the sauce to limit the temptation of over-indulging.

Enjoy your meal and eat slowly. Ask to have the plate removed when you feel full. Eat only half of the portion or share it with a friend. You can always ask for a bag to go and enjoy the leftovers later. It will be an excellent lunch meal. You can also ask for half of the meal to be held in the kitchen until you are through with your meal. Once again, just remove the temptation!

Make Healthier Beverage Choices: Have a non-caloric beverage like tea, seltzer water, water, sugar-free or diet soda. Choose a splash or orange juice or cranberry juice in some seltzer water for a fizzy surprise.

Make Healthy Dessert Choices: Have a cup of coffee, cappuccino, or some herbal tea with a sugar substitute or no sugar with some skim milk. Order a dessert for everyone at the table to enjoy. Order some berries or mixed fruit.

Slow Down: Try eating slower and chewing your food more thoroughly. Put your utensils down between mouthfuls to help slow you down. It will also give you time for satiety to kick in.

Prevent yourself from going to all you can eat buffets. This is a nightmare for portion control. Don't tempt fate if you're just beginning your new diet program. Choose a smaller plate when you go to the buffet. You can also choose a normal size plate or fill it half full of veggies or salad.

Restaurant Options for the Mediterranean Diet Plan

These are just a few of the ways to enjoy your outing:

McDonald's: These are some of the healthy choices:

- Apple Dippers with a low-fat caramel dip or a yogurt parfait.
- Caesar Salad & Grilled Chicken
- Bacon Ranch Salad & Grilled Chicken

Subway: Choose a Subway Club Salad, Savory Turkey Breast Salad, or many others. You can choose any 6-inch sub with the following ingredients:

- Roast Beef
- Oven Roasted Chicken Breast
- Savory Turkey Breast
- Subway Club
- Savory Turkey Breast & Ham
- Ham
- Honey Mustard Ham
- Sweet Onion Chicken Teriyaki

Taco Bell: You can cut the fats in your food by 25% if you order any of these items using the Fresco style which will provide 350 calories or less and under ten grams of fat. These are just two of your choices:

- Beef Soft Taco: 160-200 calories
- Burrito Supreme for 390-420 calories. The Fresco burrito is 340-350 calories.

Pyramid of the Mediterranean Diet

Overall: Yes, Plenty of water is at the head of the list for every day!

Your Monthly Allowance:

- 4 Servings - Red meat

Your Weekly Allowance:

- **3 Servings**: Eggs - Potatoes - Sweets
- **3-4 Servings**: Nuts, Olives, Pulses
- **7-14 tbsp.**: Olive oil
- **4 Servings**: Legumes - Poultry
- **5-6 Servings**: Fish

Your Daily Allowance:

- **3 Servings**: Fruit - Dairy Products
- **6 Servings**: Vegetables
- **8 Servings**: Non-refined products and cereals (brown rice, whole grain bread, etc.)

Olive Oil: Acts as a major added lipid

Learn Portion Control

These are some general guidelines so you can better calculate the serving sizes for your meal planning needs:

- **Meat**: 2.1 ounces of fish or lean meat

- **Potatoes**: 3.5 ounces

- **Vegetables**: 1 cup of raw - leafy veggies or .5 cup of all others

- **Dairy**: 1 cup of yogurt or 1 cup of milk; 1.1 ounces of cheese

- **Eggs**: 1 egg

- **Grains:** .5 cup cooked rice or pasta; 1 slice of bread is almost 1 ounce

- **Nuts**: 30 grams (1.1 ounces): Sprinkled on foods for flavor or as a snack

- **Legumes**: 100 grams (1 cup) of dry cooked beans

- **Fruit**: 1 orange, 1 apple, 1 banana, 1 ounce of grapes, 7.1 ounces of watermelon or other melons

- **Wine**: 125 ml or about a 4.2-ounce glass of a regular strength red wine

Chapter 4: Exercise Is Essential

Your weight will depend on the amount of energy your body burns and how much energy you consume from beverage and food products. Before we begin, let's discuss a little about the science of how weight loss works. In short, if you consume more calories (more food) than your body can use; you add on the pounds. The excess or extra energy is converted to fat and is stored in your body. If the ratio of the number of calories that you ingest equals the amount your body is using; your weight will remain stable or unchanged.

However, if you consume fewer calories than your body can use; you will lose weight. It requires your body to 'tap into' the stored body fat to obtain the additional energy needed. In one pound of fat, you receive about 3,500 calories. If you lower the calories by eating better on the plan; you can cut the calories by about 500 calories daily which can result in one pound of weight loss weekly.

This is the beauty of the Mediterranean way of eating healthier; you don't want to drop the pounds too quickly, but you could with a new eating pattern. If you lose more than one kilogram or about 2.2 pounds; instead of losing the unwanted fat, you might be losing muscle tissue instead. In short, that's why you need to get more exercise and eat fewer calories.

How to Proceed

It is important to increase your physical activities for about thirty minutes each day as part of your new diet regimen. You can begin slowly with a walk, go for a swim, go for a bicycle ride, or go for a jog.

If you have any other risk factors such as smoking; maybe it is time to consider breaking the habit. Have your blood pressure frequently checked, so you know your diet plan is working for you.

Research has shown if you have a strict Mediterranean diet, and exercise regularly; you can keep your weight under control. With the filling menus you will be planning, you won't be hungry and end up with unwanted calories or inches around your waistline. After all, a sedentary lifestyle is a major contributing factor to obesity.

Begin & Maintain a Regular Exercise Program

You should consider exercising 30-60 minutes daily as an integral part of healthy living choices. Regular physical activity benefits your strength, mood, and balance. If you've been living a more sedentary lifestyle, it's vital for you to speak with your doctor about a safe exercise regimen. Make sure you start off slow. Progressively pick up the pace and regularity of your workouts.

Physicians suggest patients suffering from pressure issues should engage in dynamic, moderate-intensity, aerobic exercise for a minimum of 1/2 hour each day. You can enjoy jogging, walking, swimming, or cycling on five days each week. Start using a pedometer and set a new goal of activity using a base of 10,000 steps daily. Get started with a group of friends and walk or start a workout group.

Plan Walking With the Family. Start making Saturday morning your 'walk day' for the entire family. Take a Sunday walk instead of taking a Sunday drive. Walk instead of driving, whenever you can. After the evening meal, go for a walk with the family. Make it a daily habit.

Go out Of Your Way to Walk: If you take a bus, make an early stop, and walk part of the way. When you go shopping, park a few aisles further away, and take a walk. While you are window shopping, go for a brisk walk in the mall. If you have a choice of an elevator or the stairs; burn a few calories!

These are a few examples of how to *moderately* burn those extra calories:

- Housework - 60 min.
- Cycling - 6 min.
- Walking - 15 min.
- Running - 10 min.
- Swimming laps - 20 min.

Regular exercise can help strengthen your muscles and keep them flexible. One huge benefit is its ability to help improve your sense of well-being and control your weight. However, cardiac patients should avoid running and white training without getting professional advice.

Try a few of these moves:

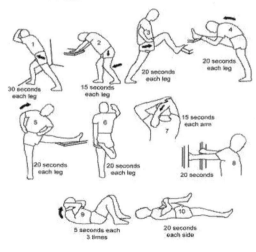

When you reach a goal, the important thing is to reward yourself.

Avoid distractions and relax. Leave the television off and take a leisurely a half-hour walk to remove the stress of the day. Just stay busy and your future will be much brighter with a much healthier outlook.

Chapter 5: 4-Week Meal Plan

Each of these daily plans is arranged according to the season. You can begin anywhere, but many of the items are calculated (when possible) according to temperatures and seasons in the United States.

Week 1: Summer Menu Option

Day 1:

Breakfast: Broccoli Cheese Omelet: 4 servings (+) 229 calories
Lunch: Arugula Salad: 4 servings (+) 257 calories
Dinner: Feta Chicken Burgers: 6 servings (+) 356 calories
Snack or Dessert: Strawberry Rhubarb Smoothie: 1 serving (+) 295 calories

Day 2:

Breakfast: Egg White Scramble with Cherry Tomatoes & Spinach:
4 servings (+) 142 calories
Lunch: Cucumber Salad: 4 servings (+) 68 calories
Dinner: Baked Salmon with Dill: 4 servings (+) 251 calories
Snack or Dessert: Fruit - Veggie & Cheese Board: 4 servings (+) 213 calories

Day 3:

Breakfast: Peanut Butter & Banana Greek Yogurt Bowl:
4 servings (+) 370 calories
Lunch: Feta Frittata: 2 servings (+) 203 calories
Dinner: Italian Chicken Skillet: 4 servings (+) 515 calories
Snack or Dessert: Honey Lime Fruit Salad: 8 servings (+) 115 calories

Day 4:

Breakfast: Poached Eggs: 2 servings (+) 72 calories
Lunch: Grecian Pasta Chicken Skillet: 4 servings (+) 373 calories
Dinner: Rosemary Thyme Lamb Chops: 4 servings (+) 231 calories
Snack or Dessert: Garlic Garbanzo Bean Spread: 2 tbsp. servings (+) 114 calories (Add your favorite crackers.)

Day 5:

Breakfast: Prosciutto - Lettuce - Tomato & Avocado Sandwiches: 4 servings (+) 240 calories
Lunch: Insalata Caprese II Salad: 6 servings (+) 311 calories
Dinner: Tomato Feta Salad: 4 servings (+) 121 calories
Snack or Dessert: Watermelon Cubes: 16 servings (+) 7 calories

Day 6:

Breakfast: Scrambled Eggs with Spinach – Tomato & Feta: 1-2
servings (+) 216 calories
Lunch: Quinoa Fruit Salad: 4 servings (+) 206 calories
Dinner: Lemon Chicken Skewers: 6 servings (+) 219 calories
Snack or Dessert: Chilled Dark Chocolate Fruit Kebabs: 6 servings (+) 254 calories

Day 7:

Breakfast: Spinach Omelet: 4 servings (+) 295 calories
Lunch: Shrimp Orzo Salad: 8 servings (+) 397 calories
Dinner: Summertime Mixed Spice Burgers: 6 servings (+) 192 calories

Snack or Dessert: Mango Pear Smoothie: 1 serving (+) 293 calories

Week 2

Day 8:

Breakfast: Avocado & Egg Breakfast Sandwich: 2 servings (+) 309 calories
Lunch: Avocado & Tuna Tapas: 4 servings (+) 294 calories
Dinner: Slow Cooked Lemon Chicken: 6 servings (+) 336 calories
Snack or Dessert: Honey Nut Granola: 6 servings (+) 337 calories

Day 9:

Breakfast: Baked Ricotta & Pears: 4 servings (+) 312 calories
Lunch: Roasted Tomato Pita Pizzas: 6 servings (+) 259 calories
Dinner: Herb-Crusted Halibut: 4 servings (+) 273 calories
Snack or Dessert: Kale Chips: 4 servings (+) 56 calories

Day 10:

Breakfast: Feta & Quinoa Egg Muffins: 12 servings (+) 113 calories
Lunch: Greek Lentil Soup: 4 servings (+) 357 calories
Dinner: Braised Chicken & Artichoke Hearts: 4 servings (+) 707 calories
Snack or Dessert: Walnut & Date Smoothie: 2 servings (+) 385 calories

Day 11:

Breakfast: Mashed Chickpea - Feta & Avocado Toast: 4 servings (+) 337 calories
Lunch: Cannellini Bean Lettuce Wraps: 4 servings (+) 211 calories
Dinner: Marinated Tuna Steak: 4 servings (+) 200 calories
Snack or Dessert: Italian Vanilla Greek Yogurt Affogato:

4 servings (+) 270 calories

Day 12:

Breakfast: Ham & Egg Cups: 8 servings (+) 145 calories
Lunch: Stuffed Bell Peppers: 6 servings (+) 210 calories
Dinner: Penne with Shrimp: 8 servings (+) 385 calories
Snack or Dessert: Strawberry Greek Frozen Yogurt: 1 quart (+) 86 calories

Day 13:

Breakfast: Pumpkin Pancakes: 6 servings (+) 278 calories
Lunch: Mushroom Risotto: 4 servings (+) 322 calories
Dinner: Pan Seared Salmon: 4 servings (+) 371 calories
Snack or Dessert: Spiced Sweet Roasted Red Pepper Hummus: 8 servings (+) 64 calories (Add your favorite veggies.)

Day 14:

Breakfast: Scrambled Eggs With Goat Cheese & Roasted Pepper: 4 servings (+) 201 calories
Lunch: Stuffed Sweet Potatoes: 4 servings (+) 142.5 calories
Dinner: Speedy Tilapia With Avocado & Red Onion: 4 servings (+) 200 calories
Snack or Dessert: Honey Rosemary Almonds: 6 servings (+) 149 calories

Week 3

Day 15:

Breakfast: Christmas Breakfast Sausage Casserole: 8 servings (+) 377 calories
Lunch: Chicken Marrakesh: 8 servings (+) 290 calories
Dinner: Nicoise-Style Tuna Salad With Olives & White Beans: 4 servings (+) 548 calories
Snack or Dessert: Chocolate Avocado Pudding: 4 servings (+) 295.3 calories

Day 16:

Breakfast: Barley Porridge: 4 servings (+) 354 calories
Lunch: Cucumber Dill Greek Yogurt Salad: 6 servings (+) 49.6 calories
Dinner: Mediterranean Pork Chops: 4 servings (+) 161 calories
Snack or Dessert: *Banana Sour Cream Bread*: 32 servings (+) 263 calories

Day 17:

Breakfast: French Toast Delight: 12 servings (+) 123 calories
Lunch: Chicken & White Bean Soup: 6 servings (+) 248 calories
Dinner: Beef Cacciatore: 6 servings (+) 510 calories
Snack or Dessert: Chia Greek Yogurt Pudding: 4 servings (+) 263 calories

Day 18:

Breakfast: Crustless Spinach Quiche: 6 servings (+) 309 calories
Lunch: Italian Tuna Sandwiches: 4 servings (+) 347 calories
Dinner: Sweet Sausage Marsala: 6 servings (+) 509 calories
Snack or Dessert: Italian Apple Olive Oil Cake: 12 serv-

ings (+) 294 calories

Day 19:

Breakfast: Fruit Bulgur Breakfast Bowl: 6 servings (+) 301 calories
Lunch: Dill Salmon Salad Wraps: 6 servings (+) 336 calories
Dinner: Beef With Artichokes - Slow Cooker: 6 servings (+) 416 calories
Snack or Dessert: Maple Vanilla Baked Pears: 4 servings (+) 103.9 calories

Day 20:

Breakfast: Marinara Eggs With Parsley: 6 servings (+) 122 calories
Lunch: Fried Rice With Spinach - Peppers & Artichokes: 4 servings (+) 244 calories
Dinner: Slow Cooked Roasted Turkey Breast: 8 servings (+) 333 calories
Snack or Dessert: Olive Oil Chocolate Chip Cookies: 24 servings (+) 187 calories

Day 21:

Breakfast: Greek Yogurt Bowl With Peanut Butter & Bananas: 4 servings (+) 370 calories
Lunch: Mediterranean Bean Salad: 4 servings (+) 329 calories
Dinner: Spanish Moroccan Fish: 12 servings (+) 268 calories
Snack or Dessert: Mediterranean Flatbread: 6 servings (+) 450 calories

Week 4:

Day 22:

**Breakfast: Greek Yogurt Breakfast Parfait with Roasted

Grapes: 4 servings (+) 300 calories
Lunch: Chicken & Veggie Wraps: 4 servings (+) 278 calories
Dinner: Salmon With Warm Tomato-Olive Salad: 4 servings (+) 433 calories
Snack or Dessert: Roasted Peaches & Blueberries: 4 servings (+) 45.7 calories

Day 23:

Breakfast: Mediterranean Egg - Pepper & Mushroom Cup: 12 servings (+) 67 calories
Lunch: Greek Shrimp Farro Bowl: 2 servings (+) 428 calories
Dinner: Mussels With Olives & Potatoes: 4 servings (+) 345 calories
Snack or Dessert: Date Wraps: 16 servings (+) 35 calories

Day 24:

Breakfast: Artichoke Frittata: 4 servings (+) 199 calories
Lunch: Goat Cheese Salad: 4 servings (+) 322 calories
Dinner: Grilled Salmon: 4 servings (+) 214 calories
Snack or Dessert: Pistachio No-Bake Snack Bars: 8 servings (+) 220 calories

Day 25:

Breakfast: Greek Yogurt Pancakes: 6 servings (+) 258 calories
Lunch: Escarole with Garlic: 4 servings (+) 66 calories
Dinner: Chicken Thighs With Artichokes & Sun-Dried Tomatoes: 6 servings (+) 169 calories
Snack or Dessert: Mango Mousse: 4 servings (+) 358 calories

Day 26:

Breakfast: Overnight Blueberry French Toast: 10 servings (+) 485 calories

Lunch: Chickpea Salad: 4 servings (+) 163 calories

Dinner: Greek Honey & Lemon Pork Chops: 4 servings (+) 257 calories

Snack or Dessert: Yogurt & Olive Oil Brownies: 12 servings (+) 150 calories

Day 27:

Breakfast: Greek Egg Frittata: 6 servings (+) 107 calories
Lunch: Mediterranean Tuna Salad: 4 servings (+) 328 calories
Dinner: Greek Salad Tacos: 4 servings (+) 466 calories
Snack or Dessert: Sautéed Apricots: 4 servings (+) 207 calories

Day 28:

Breakfast: Roasted Asparagus Prosciutto & Egg: 4 servings (+) 199 calories
Lunch: Pasta With Sausage & Escarole: 4 servings (+) 333 calories
Dinner: Grilled Lamb Chops With Mint: 6 servings (+) 238 calories
Snack or Dessert: Almond-Stuffed Dates: 1 serving (+) 149 calories

Consider Adding Meal Prep for the Mediterranean Plan

Now that you have a great meal plan, you may decide it's time to consider doing a little bit of meal prep. This is especially true if you are just cooking for one or two people. Most recipes have four servings or more in them. You can start small by using a few essential products. You can save a ton of money by storing the extra food in the freezer to use at a later time when you just don't have time to prepare a meal from scratch.

Do you want to prepare all of the chicken, pork or other meal selections one night and the veggies the next night? Or: Do you want to cook each meal individually but in bulk? Either way, these are a few of the items to help you begin:

- Ziploc-type freezer bags
- Mason Jars – Pint or quart sized
- Rubbermaid Stackable - Glad Containers

The main thing to remember is to purchase items that are stackable, reusable, BPA-free, freezer safe, and microwavable. Choose a time when you won't be interrupted. Try to find meat and dairy that has an expiration date for as far in the future as possible. These choices will tend to remain fresh and last longer. This also applies to the "sell by" dates. The further in the future, either of these dates is, the surer you can be that the food is going to last the week. Dice or chop your own meats and vegetables and stop paying for the convenience.

Look Ahead For Emergencies:

- Prepare and freeze plenty of healthy fruits and yogurt into a delicious smoothie for the entire week. Enjoy one for breakfast or any time you have the craving. Chop your veggies in advance.

- As you prep, include lean proteins for the weekends in a container for a quick grab and go snack or luncheon for a weekend journey.

- Purchase foods in bulk to be used for taco meats, breakfast burritos, fajita fillings, soups, egg muffins, and so much more.

You will help eliminate stress. You will also love the fact that these foods will be ready when you are!

Chapter 6: Recipes for the Summer

Breakfast for Summer

Broccoli & Cheese Omelet

Serving Yields: 4
Nutritional Calorie Count: 229

Ingredients Needed:
- Fresh broccoli florets - 2.5 cups
- Large eggs - 6
- 2% milk - .25 cup
- Salt - .5 tsp.
- Pepper - .25 tsp.
- Grated Romano cheese - .33 cup
- Sliced pitted Greek olives - 33 cup
- Olive oil - 1 tbsp.
- To Garnish: Shaved Romano cheese & Minced fresh parsley
- Also Needed: 10-inch ovenproof skillet

Preparation Instructions:
1. Set the oven temperature to broil.
2. Place a steamer basket in a saucepan in about 1 inch of water. Toss the broccoli into the basket. Wait for it to boil.
3. Lower the heat to simmer for four to six minutes with a lid on.
4. Whisk the eggs, milk, salt, and pepper. Fold in the broccoli, olives, and grated cheese.
5. Prepare the skillet using the medium heat setting and add the oil. Fold in the egg mixture and cook for 6 minutes.
6. Place the skillet in the oven approximately 3-4 inches from the heat. Bake for 2-4 minutes or until the eggs are set.

7. Transfer to the countertop to cool for about 5 minutes.
8. Slice into wedges. Sprinkle with the parsley and shaved cheese.

Egg White Scramble with Cherry Tomatoes & Spinach

Serving Yields: 4
Nutritional Calorie Count: 142

Ingredients Needed:

- Olive oil - 1 tbsp.
- Eggs - 1 whole & 10 egg whites
- Black pepper - .25 tsp.
- Salt - .5 tsp.
- Minced garlic clove - 1
- Halved cherry tomatoes - 2 cups
- Packed fresh baby spinach - 2 cups
- Light cream or Half & Half - .5 cup
- Finely grated parmesan cheese - .25 cup

Preparation Instructions:

1. Whisk the eggs, pepper, salt, and milk.
2. Prepare a skillet using the med-hi heat setting.
3. Toss in the garlic when the pan is hot. Sauté for approximately 30 seconds.
4. Pour in the tomatoes and spinach. Continue sautéing for one additional minute. The tomatoes should be softened and the spinach wilted.
5. Add the egg mixture into the pan using the medium heat setting. Fold the egg gently as it cooks for about two to three minutes.
6. Remove from the burner, and sprinkle with a sprinkle of cheese.

Peanut Butter & Banana Greek Yogurt Bowl

Serving Yields: 4
Nutritional Calorie Count: 370

Ingredients Needed:

- Medium bananas - 2
- Flaxseed meal - .25 cup
- Nutmeg - 1 tsp.
- Peanut butter - .25 cup
- Greek yogurt - vanilla - 4 cups

Preparation Instructions:

1. Peel and slice the bananas. Divide the yogurt amongst four serving dishes. Top each one off with sliced bananas.
2. Microwave the peanut butter for 30 to 40 seconds until completely melted.
3. Drizzle the peanut butter over the banana slices and sprinkle with the flaxseed meal. Top it off with the nutmeg and serve.

Poached Eggs

Serving Yields: 2
Nutritional Calorie Count: 72

Ingredients Needed:

- Salt - .5 tsp.
- Champagne vinegar - 1 tsp.
- Fresh eggs - 2

Preparation Instructions:

1. Prepare a saucepan with cold water and bring it to a boil using the medium temperature setting. Stir in the salt and vinegar.
2. Break each of the eggs into a ramekin. Place it close to the water and slide it out of the dish. Simmer until set.
3. Use a slotted spoon to lift it from the pan to help prevent sticking. Continue cooking until the yolk is runny and the white is cooked or about six minutes.
4. Prepare a container with ice water. Transfer the eggs from the pan to the bowl of ice water (It slows and stops the cooking process.)
5. Remove from the pan and drain on a paper towel before serving.

Prosciutto – Lettuce – Tomato & Avocado Sandwiches

Serving Yields: 4
Nutritional Calorie Count: 240

Ingredients Needed:

- Whole grain or whole wheat bread slices - 8
- Freshly ground black pepper - .25 tsp.
- Ripe avocado - 1 cut in half
- Kosher or sea salt - .25 tsp.
- Romaine lettuce - 4 full leaves
- Large ripe tomato - 1
- Prosciutto - 2 oz. - 8 thin slices

Preparation Instructions:

1. Tear the lettuce leaves into 8 pieces (total). Slice the tomato into two 8 rounds. Toast the bread and place it on a plate.
2. Use a spoon to remove the avocado flesh from the skin. Add it to a bowl. Sprinkle with the salt and pepper.
3. Whisk or gently mash the avocado until it's creamy. Spread over the bread.
4. Make one sandwich. Take a slice of avocado toast; top it with a lettuce leaf, a prosciutto slice, and a tomato slice. Top with another slice of lettuce tomato and continue. Repeat until all ingredients are made for four sandwiches.

Scrambled Eggs with Spinach – Tomato & Feta

Serving Yields: 1-2
Nutritional Calorie Count: 216

Ingredients Needed:

- Tomato – .5 of 1 - .33 cup
- Vegetable oil - 1 tbsp.
- Baby spinach - 1 cup
- Eggs - 3
- Pepper and salt - as desired
- Feta cheese - 2 tbsp.

Preparation Instructions:

1. Remove the seeds and dice the tomatoes. Cut the feta into cubes.
2. Warm up a skillet using the medium heat setting.
3. Sauté the spinach and tomatoes.
4. Once the spinach has wilted, whisk and stir in the eggs.
5. Scramble until done and give it a dusting of the salt and pepper.

Spinach Omelet

Serving Yields: 4
Nutritional Calorie Count: 295

Ingredients Needed:

- Olive oil - 3 tbsp.
- Small onion - 1
- Garlic clove - 1
- Large tomatoes - 4
- Eggs - 8
- Black pepper - .25 tsp.
- Fine sea salt - 1 tsp.
- Feta cheese - 2 oz.
- Flat leaf parsley - 1 tbsp.

Preparation Instructions:

1. Core and chop the tomatoes, parsley, and onion.
2. Warm up the oven to reach 400° Fahrenheit.
3. Pour the oil into an ovenproof skillet using high heat. Toss in the onions. Sauté until softened (5-7 min.).
4. Pour in the tomatoes, garlic, salt, and pepper.
5. Sauté for five more minutes and add the whisked eggs. Stir and cook for 3 to 5 minutes. When the bottom is set, put the skillet into the hot oven. Continue cooking for 5 additional minutes.
6. Transfer to the countertop and top it off with the parsley and feta. Serve warm.

Lunch Options for the Summer

Arugula Salad

Serving Yields: 4
Nutritional Calorie Count: 257

Ingredients Needed:

- Arugula leaves - 4 cups
- Cherry tomatoes - 1 cup
- Pine nuts - .25 cup
- Rice vinegar - 1 tbsp.
- Grape seed or olive oil - 2 tbsp.
- Pepper & Salt - to your liking
- Grated parmesan cheese - .25 cup
- Large avocado - 1 sliced

Preparation Instructions:

1. Rinse and dry the arugula leaves, grate the cheese, and slice the cherry tomatoes into halves. Peel and slice the avocado.
2. Combine the arugula, pine nuts, tomatoes, oil, vinegar, and cheese.
3. Sprinkle with a dusting of pepper and salt as desired.
4. Cover and toss to mix. Portion onto plates with the avocado slices, and enjoy.

Cucumber Salad

Serving Yields: 4
Nutritional Calorie Count: 68

Ingredients Needed:

- Cucumbers - 5-6
- Plain Greek yogurt - 8 oz.
- Garlic cloves - 2
- Oregano - 1 tsp.
- Fresh mint - 1 tbsp.
- Black pepper and Fine sea salt - .125 tsp. each

Preparation Instructions:

1. Use a sharp paring knife to slice the cucumbers. Mince the mint and garlic.
2. Mix the oregano, mint, garlic, yogurt, with the cucumbers in a mixing bowl. Sprinkle the cucumbers with the pepper and salt.
3. Place in the refrigerator for approximately one hour before your meal.

Feta Frittata

Serving Yields: 2
Nutritional Calorie Count: 203

Ingredients Needed:

- Green onion - 1
- Small garlic clove - 1
- Large eggs - 2
- Egg substitute - .5 cup
- Crumbled feta cheese - divided - 4 tbsp.
- Plum tomato - .33 cup
- Avocado slices - 4 thin
- Reduced-fat sour cream - 2 tbsp.
- Also Needed: 6-inch nonstick skillet

Preparation Instructions:

1. Thinly slice the onion and mince the garlic clove, chop the tomato, and peel the avocado before slicing.
2. Warm up the pan using the medium temperature setting and lightly spritz it with cooking oil.
3. Whisk the egg substitute, eggs, and three tablespoons of the feta cheese.
4. Add the egg mixture into the pan. Cover and simmer for 4 to 6 minutes.
5. Sprinkle with the rest of the feta cheese and tomato. Cover and continue cooking until the eggs are set or about 2 to 3 more minutes.
6. Let it rest for about 5 minutes before cutting it into halves. Serve with the avocado and sour cream.

Grecian Pasta Chicken Skillet

Serving Yields: 4 - 1.5 cups each
Nutritional Calorie Count: 373

Ingredients Needed:

- Reduced-sodium chicken broth - 1 can - 14.5 oz.
- Diced tomatoes undrained - no salt added - 1 can - 14.5 oz.
- Chicken breast - cut into 1-inch pieces - .75 lb.
- Water or white wine - .5 cup
- Garlic - 1 clove
- Dried oregano - .5 tsp.
- Multigrain thin spaghetti - 4 oz.
- Marinated and quartered artichoke hearts - 7.5 oz. jar
- Roasted sweet bell pepper strips - .25 cup
- Sliced ripe olives - .25 cup
- Baby spinach - 2 cups
- Chopped green onion - 1
- Fresh parsley - 2 tbsp.
- Lemon juice - 2 tbsp.
- Grated lemon zest - .5 tsp.
- Olive oil - 1 tbsp.
- Pepper - .5 tsp.
- Optional: Crumbled reduced-fat feta cheese to your liking

Preparation Instructions:

1. Drain and coarsely chop the artichoke hearts.
2. Combine the water/wine, chicken, garlic, oregano, chicken broth, and tomatoes in a large skillet.
3. Toss in the spaghetti and boil for 5-7 minutes. Simmer until the pink is removed from the chicken.
4. Stir in the spinach, pepper, oil, parsley, green onion, olives, red peppers, and the juice and zest of lemon.
5. Simmer for another 2-3 minutes or until the spinach is

wilted.

6. Sprinkle with the cheese and serve.

Insalata Caprese II Salad

Serving Yields: 6
Nutritional Calorie Count: 311

Ingredients Needed:

- Large ripened tomato - .25-inches thick - 4
- Mozzarella cheese - .25-inches thick - 1 lb.
- Fresh basil leaves - .33 cup
- Extra-virgin olive oil - 3 tbsp.
- Fine sea salt - as desired
- Freshly cracked black pepper - as desired

Preparation Instructions:

1. Prepare the salad by alternating and overlapping tomato slices with mozzarella cheese and the basil leaves.
2. Spritz with the olive oil and dust with a portion of the pepper and salt. Serve.

Quinoa Fruit Salad

Serving Yields: 4
Nutritional Calorie Count: 206

Ingredients Needed:

- Raw honey - 2 tbsp.
- Fresh strawberries - 1 cup
- Fresh lime juice - 2 tbsp.
- Cooked quinoa - 1 cup
- Diced mango - 1
- Fresh blackberries - 1 cup
- Diced peach - 1
- Fresh basil - 1 tsp.
- Kiwi - 2

Preparation Instructions:

1. Slice the strawberries and dice the peach and mango.
2. Combine the basil, honey, and lime juice.
3. In another bowl, mix the mango, kiwi, peach, blackberries, quinoa, and the strawberries.
4. Stir in the honey mixture and toss well before serving.

Shrimp Orzo Salad

Serving Yields: 8
Nutritional Calorie Count: 397 - per 1.5 cup serving

Ingredients Needed:

- Orzo pasta - 16 oz. 1 pkg.
- Cooked shrimp - .75 lb.
- Water-packed artichoke hearts - 14 oz. can
- Sweet red pepper - 1 cup
- Red onion - .75 cup
- Green pepper - 1 cup
- Pitted Greek olives - .5 cup
- Freshly minced parsley - .5 cup
- Freshly chopped dill - .33 cup
- Greek vinaigrette - .75 cup

Preparation Instructions:

1. Peel and devein the shrimp and cook. Slice each one into thirds (31-40-count). Finely chop the onions and peppers.
2. Prepare the orzo according to the package instructions. Drain and rinse the orzo with cold water. Drain well.
3. Combine the shrimp, orzo, olives, herbs, and veggies.
4. Sprinkle with vinaigrette and toss to coat.
5. Refrigerate and cover until ready to serve.
6. Serve as a delicious side salad.

Dinner Specialties for the Summer

Baked Salmon with Dill

Serving Yields: 4
Nutritional Calorie Count: 251

Ingredients Needed:

- Salmon fillets - 4- 6 oz. portions - 1-inch thick
- Finely chopped fresh dill - 1.5 tbsp.
- Black pepper -.125 tsp.
- Kosher salt - .5 tsp.
- Lemon wedges - 4

Preparation Instructions:

1. Warm up the oven to reach 350° Fahrenheit.
2. Grease a baking tin with a spritz of cooking oil spray and add the fish.
3. Lightly spritz the fish with the spray along with a shake of the salt, pepper, and dill.
4. Bake for ten minutes or until the fish is easily flaked with a fork.
5. Serve with the lemon wedges.

Feta Chicken Burgers

Serving Yields: 6
Nutritional Calorie Count: 356 with 1 tbsp. sauce

Ingredients Needed:

- Reduced-fat mayonnaise - .25 cup
- Finely chopped cucumber - .25 cup
- Black pepper - .25 tsp.
- Garlic powder - 1 tsp.
- Chopped roasted sweet red pepper - .5 cup
- Greek seasoning - .5 tsp.
- Lean ground chicken - 1.5 lb.
- Crumbled feta cheese - 1 cup
- Whole wheat burger buns - 6 toasted

Preparation Instructions:

1. Warm up the broiler to the oven ahead of time. Combine the mayonnaise and cucumber together. Set aside.
2. Combine all of the seasonings and the red pepper for the burgers. Work in the chicken and the cheese. Shape into 6 - ½-inch thick patties.
3. Broil the burgers approximately four inches from the heat source. It should take about 3-4 minutes on each side until the thermometer reaches 165° Fahrenheit.
4. Serve on the buns with the cucumber sauce. Top it off with tomato and lettuce if desired and serve.

Italian Chicken Skillet

Serving Yields: 4
Nutritional Calorie Count: 515

Ingredients Needed:

- Olive oil - 1 tbsp.
- Chicken breast halves - 4
- Garlic - 2 cloves
- Red cooking wine - .5 cup
- Italian style diced tomatoes - 28 oz. can
- Seashell pasta - 8 oz.
- Freshly chopped spinach - 5 oz.
- Shredded mozzarella cheese - 1 cup

Preparation Instructions:

1. Warm up a large skillet and add the oil.
2. Add the chicken and simmer for about five to eight minutes.
3. Pour in the diced tomatoes and wine. Let it come to a boil using the high heat setting.
4. Stir in the pasta. Leave the top off and continue cooking. Stir occasionally until the shells are thoroughly cooked (10 min. after the pasta starts boiling).
5. Spread the spinach over top of the pasta and cover. The spinach should be ready in about 5 minutes.
6. Sprinkle with the cheese and simmer for another five minutes or until the cheese is bubbling.

Lemon Chicken Skewers

Serving Yields: 6
Nutritional Calorie Count: 219

Ingredients Needed:

- Olive oil - .25 cup
- Lemon juice - 3 tbsp.
- White wine vinegar - 1 tbsp.
- Grated lemon zest - 2 tsp.
- Salt - 1 tsp.
- Dried oregano - .25 tsp.
- Freshly cracked black pepper - .25 tsp.
- Sugar - .5 tsp.
- Zucchini - 3 medium - 1.5-inch slices
- Minced garlic - 2 cloves
- Medium onions - 3 into wedges
- Cherry tomatoes - 12
- Chicken breasts - 1.5 lb.

Preparation Instructions:

1. Cut the zucchini in half lengthwise and slice into 1.5-inch slices.
2. Peel the onions and cut into wedges. Zest the lemon. Cut the chicken into 1.5-inch pieces.
3. Prepare the marinade; combine the sugar, pepper, oregano, salt, lemon zest, vinegar, lemon juice, and oil - reserving .25 cup for basting.
4. Fold in the chicken and toss to cover.
5. Add the rest of the marinade in a mixing container and add the tomatoes, onions, and zucchini. Cover and place in the fridge overnight (for best results) or a minimum of four hours.
6. When ready to cook, drain and trash the marinade.
7. Soak the wooden skewers in water.

8. Thread the chicken and veggies onto the soaked skewers.
9. Place the skewers on the grill for six minutes using the medium heat setting. It's done when poked with a fork - the juices will run clear.

Rosemary Thyme Lamb Chops

Serving Yields: 4
Nutritional Calorie Count: 231

Ingredients Needed:

- Lamb loin chops - 8 - 3 oz. each
- Salt - .25 tsp.
- Pepper - .5 tsp.
- Dijon mustard - 3 tbsp.
- Fresh rosemary - 1 tbsp.
- Garlic - 3 cloves
- Fresh thyme - 1 tbsp.

Preparation Instructions:

1. Mince the thyme and garlic.
2. Combine the mustard, garlic, rosemary, and thyme in a mixing container. Sprinkle the lamb chops with the pepper and salt.
3. Lightly grease the grill rack. Prepare the chops on the grill using the medium heat setting for 6-8 minutes. For Doneness: Med-well is 145° Fahrenheit, the medium is 140° Fahrenheit, and well-done is at 135° Fahrenheit.

Summertime Mixed Spice Burgers

Serving Yields: 6
Nutritional Calorie Count: 192

Ingredients Needed:

- Finely chopped medium onion - 1
- Freshly minced parsley - 3 tbsp.
- Clove of garlic - 1 minced
- Ground allspice - .75 tsp.
- Pepper - .75 tsp.
- Ground nutmeg - .25 tsp.
- Cinnamon - .5 tsp.
- Salt - .5 tsp.
- Fresh mint - 2 tbsp.
- 90% lean ground beef - 1.5 lb.
- Tzatziki sauce - optional

Preparation Instructions:

1. Whisk the nutmeg, salt, cinnamon, pepper, allspice, garlic cloves, minced mint, parsley, and the onion.
2. Add the beef and prepare (6) 2 by 4-inch oblong patties.
3. Use the medium heat setting to grill the patties or broil four inches from the heat source for four to six minutes per side.
4. When it's done, the meat thermometer will register 160° Fahrenheit. Serve with the sauce if desired.

Tomato Feta Salad

Serving Yields: 4
Nutritional Calorie Count: 121

Ingredients Needed:

- Balsamic vinegar - 2 tbsp.
- Freshly minced basil - 1.5 tsp. or .5 tsp. dried
- Salt -.5 tsp.
- Coarsely chopped sweet onion - .5 cup
- Olive oil - 2 tbsp.
- Cherry or grape tomatoes - 1 lb.
- Crumbled feta cheese - .25 cup.

Preparation Instructions:

1. Whisk the salt, basil, and vinegar.
2. Toss the onion into the vinegar mixture, and let it rest for about 5 minutes
3. Slice the tomatoes into halves and stir in the tomatoes, feta cheese, and oil type evenly. Serve.

Snacks for the Summer

Chilled Dark Chocolate Fruit Kebabs

Serving Yields: 6
Nutritional Calorie Count: 254

Ingredients Needed:

- Hulled strawberries - 12
- Green or red seedless grapes - 24
- Pitted cherries - 12
- Blueberries - 24
- Dark chocolate - 8 oz.

Preparation Instructions:

1. Prepare a rimmed baking sheet with a layer of parchment paper. Lay out six 12-inch skewers. Prepare the skewers with the fruit - alternating each flavor.
2. Use a microwave-safe dish to heat the chocolate on high for one minute. Stir to melt the chocolate.
3. Add the melted chocolate to a plastic sandwich bag and twist a corner. Snip the corner off of the bag to use as a pipe. Squeeze the bag to drizzle the chocolate over the kebabs.
4. Arrange the sheet in the freezer to chill for 20 minutes before serving.

Fruit – Veggie & Cheese Board

Serving Yields: 4
Nutritional Calorie Count: 213

Ingredients Needed:

- Sliced fruits - Peaches, plums, pears, or apples - 2 cups
- Finger food fruits - Figs, grapes, cherries, or berries - 2 cups
- Raw veggies cut into sticks - Cauliflower, broccoli, celery, or carrots
- Jarred, canned, or cured veggies - Artichoke hearts, roasted Peppers or 0.5 cup of olives
- Cubed cheese - Gorgonzola, goat cheese, Asiago, or feta - Approximately 6 oz. or 1 cup

Preparation Instructions:

1. Prep the produce: Wash all of the veggies and slice into bite-size pieces.
2. Arrange all of the fixings on a wooden board or a serving tray. You can also cover a baking tin with parchment paper.
3. Add small spoons and little forks for the berries and olives and a knife for cutting the cheese.
4. Serve with small individual plates and napkins.

Garlic Garbanzo Bean Spread

Serving Yields: 1.5 cups
Nutritional Calorie Count: 114 per 2 tbsp. serving

Ingredients Needed:

- Chickpeas or garbanzo beans - 1 can - 15 oz.
- Olive oil - .5 cup
- Green onion - 1 - into 3 pieces
- Lemon juice - 1 tbsp.
- Garlic cloves - 1-2 peeled
- Salt - .25 tsp.
- Freshly minced parsley - 2 tbsp.
- Baked pita chips and assorted fresh veggies
- Also Needed: Food Processor

Preparation Instructions:

1. Combine the chickpeas or garbanzo beans, oil, parsley, lemon juice, garlic, salt, and green onion.
2. Add the ingredients into the blender and process until mixed.
3. Empty into a dish and refrigerate until ready to serve.
4. Enjoy with the pita chips and veggies.

Honey Lime Fruit Salad

Serving Yields: 8
Nutritional Calorie Count: 115

Ingredients Needed:

- Sliced bananas - 2 large
- Fresh blueberries - .5 lb.
- Fresh strawberries - 1 lb.
- Honey - 2 tbsp.
- Lime - 1 juiced
- Pine nuts - .33 cup

Preparation Instructions:

1. Hull and slice the strawberries and bananas.
2. Combine the blueberries, strawberries, and bananas in a bowl.
3. Cross over with the lime juice and honey.
4. Stir well and sprinkle with the nuts before serving.

Strawberry Greek Frozen Yogurt

Serving Yields: 1 quart
Nutritional Calorie Count: 86

Ingredients Needed:

- 2% plain Greek yogurt - 3 cups
- Fresh lemon juice - .25 cup
- Sugar - 1 cup
- Vanilla - 2 tsp.
- Salt - .125 tsp.
- Sliced strawberries - 1 cup
- Also Needed: 1.5 to 2-quart ice cream maker

Preparation Instructions:

1. Whisk the vanilla, salt, lemon juice, yogurt, and sugar until creamy.
2. Place the mixture in the ice cream maker. Prepare according to the manufacturer's directions.
3. Toss in the sliced berries for the last minute of the cycle.
4. Empty into a container and freeze for two to four hours before serving.
5. Let the ice cream sit out at room temperature for about 5 to 15 minutes before serving for best results.

Watermelon Cubes

Serving Yields: 16
Nutritional Calorie Count: 7

Ingredients Needed:

- Seedless watermelon cubes - 16 - 1-inch
- Finely chopped cucumber - .33 cup
- Finely chopped red onion - 5 tsp.
- Minced fresh mint - 2 tsp.
- Lime juice - .5 - 1 tsp. lime juice
- Freshly minced cilantro - 2 tsp.

Preparation Instructions:

1. Use a measuring spoon or a small melon baller to remove the center of each of the watermelon cubes. Leave a ¼-inch shell. Use the pulp another time.
2. In a small dish, mix the remaining fixings. Spoon into the watermelon cubes and serve.

Smoothies

Mango Pear Smoothie

Serving Yields: 1
Nutritional Calorie Count: 293

Ingredients Needed:

- Plain Greek yogurt - .5 cup
- Ice cubes - 2
- Mango - .5 of 1
- Kale - 1 cup
- Ripened pear - 1

Preparation Instructions:

1. Combine each of the ingredients in a blender.
2. Mix well until thickened and smooth.
3. Serve in a chilled glass.

Strawberry Rhubarb Smoothie

Serving Yields: 1
Nutritional Calorie Count: 295

Ingredients Needed:

- Sliced strawberries - 1 cup
- Chopped rhubarb - 1 stalk
- Raw honey - 2 tbsp.
- Ice cubes - 3
- Ground cinnamon - .125 tsp.
- Plain Greek yogurt - .5 cup

Preparation Instructions:

1. Pour water into a small saucepan and add the rhubarb. Boil for 3 minutes before draining and adding to a blender.
2. Prepare the rest of the fixings and add to the blender along with the honey, yogurt, cinnamon, and ice.
3. Blend well until creamy smooth, serving a chilled glass.

Chapter 7: Recipes for the Fall & Autumn Months

Breakfast Favorites for Fall/Autumn

Avocado & Egg Breakfast Sandwich

Serving Yields: 2
Nutritional Calorie Count: 309

Ingredients Needed:

- Toasted bread slices - whole wheat - 4
- Pitted avocado - 1
- Steamed asparagus spears - 8-12
- Sliced hard-boiled egg - 1
- Olive oil - as needed
- Freshly ground pepper & coarse sea salt - as desired
- Optional: Dijon mustard

Preparation Instructions:

1. Peel and mash the avocado. Toast the bread.
2. Prepare the sandwich by using the mustard with a layer of the avocado.
3. Add the asparagus spears and eggs.
4. Give it a drizzle of oil along with some salt and pepper. Close and serve.

Baked Ricotta & Pears

Serving Yields: 4
Nutritional Calorie Count: 312

Ingredients Needed:

- Ricotta cheese - whole-milk - 16 oz. container
- Large eggs - 2
- White whole wheat flour - .25 cup
- Sugar - 1 tbsp.
- Nutmeg - .25 tsp.
- Diced pear - 1
- Water - 2 tbsp.
- Vanilla extract - 1 tsp.
- Honey - 1 tbsp.
- Also Needed: 4 - 6 oz. ramekins

Preparation Instructions:

1. Heat up the oven to reach 400° Fahrenheit.
2. Lightly spray the ramekins with a spritz of cooking oil spray.
3. Whisk the flour, nutmeg, vanilla, sugar, eggs, and the ricotta together in a large mixing container.
4. Spoon the ingredients into the dishes. Bake for 20 to 25 minutes. The ricotta should be set. Take it out of the oven. Let it cool slightly.
5. In a saucepan, using the medium temperature setting, add the cored and diced pear into the water for about 10 minutes until slightly softened. Take the pan off of the burner and stir in the honey.
6. Serve the ricotta ramekins with the warm pear and enjoy.

Feta & Quinoa Egg Muffins

Serving Yields: 12
Nutritional Calorie Count: 113

Ingredients Needed:

- Cooked quinoa - 1 cup
- Chopped baby spinach - 2 cups
- Kalamata olives - .5 cup
- Tomatoes - 1 cup
- White onion - .5 cup
- Fresh oregano - 1 tbsp.
- Salt - .5 tsp.
- Olive oil - 2 tsp. (+) more for coating pans
- Eggs - 8
- Crumbled feta cheese - 1 cup
- Also Needed: 12-cup muffin tin

Preparation Instructions:

1. Warm up the oven to reach 350° Fahrenheit.
2. Lightly grease the muffin tray cups with a spritz of cooking oil.
3. Prepare a skillet using the medium heat setting and add the oil. When hot, toss in the onions and cook for two minutes.
4. Pour in the tomatoes and sauté one minute. Add the spinach and continue cooking for another minute or until the leaves have wilted.
5. Remove from the heat and add the oregano and olives. Set aside.
6. Crack the eggs into a bowl and blend using an immersion stick blender. Add the cooked veggies in with the remainder of the ingredients.
7. Stir until combined and spoon into the greased muffin cups.

8. Bake for 30 minutes until browned and the muffins are set.
9. Cool for 10 minutes.

Ham & Egg Cups

Serving Yields: 8
Nutritional Calorie Count: 145

Ingredients Needed:

- Cooked ham – deli style - 8 thin slices
- Mozzarella cheese - .25 cups or 1 oz.
- Eggs - 8
- Basil – optional - 8 tsp.
- Black pepper - as desired
- Grape or cherry tomatoes - 6 or as desired
- Also Needed: Muffin tin - 8-count

Preparation Instructions:

1. Program the oven setting to 350°F. Coat the muffin tin cups with the spray.
2. Press the ham slice into the bottom and add the cheese to each of the prepared cups. Break an egg into the cup and sprinkle with the pepper. Add the pesto, if using. Slice the tomatoes into halves, and place on each of the cups.
3. Bake 18-20 minutes. The egg whites should be set, similar to a regular poached egg. Leave them in the cups for 3-5 minutes. Then, carefully take the cups out of the tin and serve.

Mashed Chickpea – Feta & Avocado Toast

Serving Yields: 4
Nutritional Calorie Count: 337

Ingredients Needed:

- Chickpeas - 15 oz. can
- Diced feta cheese - 2 oz. - .5 cup
- Avocado - 1 pitted
- Fresh orange juice -1 tbsp. or lemon juice - 2 tsp.
- Freshly cracked black pepper - .5 tsp.
- Honey - 2 tsp.
- Multigrain toast - 4 slices

Preparation Instructions:

1. Toast the bread. Drain the chickpeas. Scoop the avocado flesh into the bowl.
2. Use a large fork or potato masher to mash them together until the mix is spreadable.
3. Pour in the lemon juice, pepper, and the feta.
4. Mix well and divide onto the four slices of toast. Drizzle with the honey and serve.

Pumpkin Pancakes

Serving Yields: 6
Nutritional Calorie Count: 278

Ingredients Needed:

- Milk - 1.5 cups
- Egg - 1
- Pumpkin puree - 1 cup
- Vegetable oil - 2 tbsp.
- Vinegar - 2 tbsp.
- Salt - .5 tsp.
- All-purpose flour - 2 cups
- Baking powder - 2 tsp.
- Ground allspice - 1 tsp.
- Brown sugar - 3 tbsp.
- Baking soda - 1 tsp.
- Cinnamon - 1 tsp.
- Ground ginger - .5 tsp.

Preparation Instructions:

1. Whisk the vinegar, oil, egg, pumpkin, and the milk together.
2. Combine the salt, ginger, cinnamon, allspice, baking soda, brown sugar, baking powder, and the flour in another bowl.
3. Stir the fixings together just enough to combine.
4. Warm up a frying pan or oiled griddle using the medium-high temperature setting.
5. Pour the batter into the griddle (for 6 servings) and brown on both sides. Serve hot.

Scrambled Eggs with Goat Cheese & Roasted Pepper

Serving Yields: 4
Nutritional Calorie Count: 201

Ingredients Needed:

- Extra-virgin olive oil - 1.5 tsp.
- Bell peppers - 1 medium pepper - 1 cup
- Garlic - 2 cloves - 1 tsp. minced
- Large eggs - 6
- Sea salt - .25 tsp.
- Water - 2 tbsp.
- Crumbled goat cheese - 2 oz. - .5 cup
- Loosely packed chopped fresh mint - 2 tbsp.

Preparation Instructions:

1. Use the medium-high heat setting to prepare a large skillet. Add the oil.
2. When hot, toss in the peppers and simmer for about five minutes. Stir in the garlic. Continue cooking for one minute.
3. Whisk the water, eggs, and salt in a mixing dish.
4. Reduce the temperature setting to med-low.
5. Pour in the egg mixture over top of the peppers. Simmer for one to two minutes until they're set on the bottom.
6. Sprinkle with the goat cheese and continue cooking for one to two more minutes. Stir until they are soft set. Garnish with the fresh mint and serve.

Lunch Options for Fall/Autumn

Avocado & Tuna Tapas

Serving Yields: 4
Nutritional Calorie Count: 294

Ingredients Needed:

- Solid white tuna packed in water - 12 oz. can
- Mayonnaise - 1 tbsp.
- Thinly sliced green onions - 3 (+) more for garnish
- Chopped red bell pepper - .5 of 1
- Garlic salt and black pepper - to taste
- Balsamic vinegar - 1 dash
- Ripe avocados - 2

Preparation Instructions:

1. Drain the tuna well. Chop the bell pepper, and thinly slice the onions. Remove the pit and slice the avocados into halves.
2. Whisk the vinegar, red pepper, onions, mayonnaise, and tuna.
3. Sprinkle with the salt and pepper.
4. Load the avocado halves with the tuna.
5. Top it off with a portion of green onions and black pepper. Serve.

Cannellini Bean Lettuce Wraps

Serving Yields: 4
Nutritional Calorie Count: 211 - 2 wraps per serving

Ingredients Needed:

- Extra-virgin olive oil - 1 tbsp.
- Red onion - .5 cup
- Tomatoes - 1 medium - .75 cup
- Freshly cracked black pepper - .25 tsp.
- Fresh curly parsley - .25 cup
- Great Northern beans or cannellini beans - 1 can - 15 oz.
- Prepared hummus - .5 cup
- Romaine lettuce leaves - 8

Preparation Instructions:

1. Drain and rinse the veggies and beans. Chop the tomatoes and onion into fine pieces.
2. Use the medium heat setting. Add the oil into a large skillet.
3. Toss in the onions and sauté for 3 minutes. Pour in the tomatoes and pepper. Simmer for three more minutes. Stir occasionally.
4. Pour in the drained beans and continue cooking for 3 additional minutes. Mix in the parsley after removing it from the burner.
5. Spread the hummus over each of the leaves of lettuce. Spread the bean mixture to the center of each leaf. Fold it over to make a wrap and serve.

Greek Lentil Soup

Serving Yields: 4
Nutritional Calorie Count: 357

Ingredients Needed:

- Brown lentils - 8 oz.
- Olive oil - .25 cup or as needed
- Minced garlic - 1 tbsp.
- Onion - 1
- Large carrot - 1
- Water - 1 quart
- Dried oregano - 1 pinch
- Crushed dried rosemary - 1 pinch
- Bay leaves - 2
- Tomato paste - 1 tbsp.
- Salt and ground black pepper - as desired
- Optional: Red wine vinegar - 1 tsp.

Preparation Instructions:

1. Mince the garlic and chop the onion and carrot.
2. Prep the lentils in a large saucepan with enough water to cover by about 1 inch. Once the beans start boiling, cook until tender or about ten minutes and drain in a colander.
3. Warm up the oil in a pan and using the medium heat setting. Toss in the onion, carrot, and garlic. Simmer approximately five minutes.
4. Pour in the water, lentils, oregano, bay leaves, and rosemary. Once boiling, reduce the temperature setting to med-low and cover. Cook for another ten minutes.
5. Sprinkle with the pepper and salt. Stir in the tomato paste.
6. Cover and simmer 30 to 40 minutes - stirring occasionally. Add water as needed.
7. When ready to serve, drizzle with the vinegar and one teaspoon of olive oil.

Mushroom Risotto

Serving Yields: 4
Nutritional Calorie Count: 322

Ingredients Needed:

- Olive oil - 2 tbsp.
- Thinly slice shallot - 1
- Large sliced mushrooms - 10
- Red wine - .5 cup
- Faro - 1 cup
- Vegetable broth - .5 cup or as needed
- Parmesan cheese - .5 cup
- Flat leaf parsley - 1 tbsp.
- Black pepper - .25 tsp.
- Fine sea salt - 1 tsp.

Preparation Instructions:

1. Place a skillet on a stovetop burner using the high heat setting.
2. Add the oil and shallot. Simmer for 3 to 5 minutes.
3. When the shallot is softened, pour in the red wine and mushrooms.
4. Add the faro. Simmer for approximately three minutes. Stir often until the broth is absorbed. Add more broth as needed. Continue until it's tender.
5. Take the skillet from the burner and add the parmesan, salt, pepper, and parsley.
6. Serve warm.

Roasted Tomato Pita Pizzas

Serving Yields: 6
Nutritional Calorie Count: 259

Ingredients Needed:

- Grape tomatoes - 2 pints or about 3 cups
- Garlic cloves - 2 minced
- Chopped fresh thyme leaves - 1 tsp. - 6 Sprigs
- Freshly cracked black pepper - .25 tsp.
- Shredded parmesan cheese - 3 oz. or .75 cup
- Kosher or sea salt - .25 tsp.
- Whole wheat pita bread - 6

Preparation Instructions:

1. Warm up the oven to reach 425° Fahrenheit.
2. Combined the tomatoes, salt, pepper, thyme, garlic, and oil. In a baking pan.
3. Roast for 10 minutes. Pull out the rack from the oven and stir the tomatoes with a wooden spoon or spatula. Mash down to soften the tomatoes and roast for another 10 minutes.
4. Prepare the pita bread with 2 tablespoons of cheese. Arrange them on a large rimmed baking sheet. Toast for the last 5 minutes of the cooking cycle.
5. Remove everything from the oven. Stir the tomatoes and spoon out about one-third of the sauce over each of the pita bread to scrvc.

Stuffed Bell Peppers

Serving Yields: 6
Nutritional Calorie Count: 210

Ingredients Needed:

- Uncooked bulgur - .5 cup
- Ground beef - 1 lb.
- Frozen chopped spinach - 10 oz. pkg.
- Medium red bell peppers - 3
- Grated zucchini - 2 cups
- Chopped tomatoes - 29 oz.
- Minced white onion - 1 cup
- Salt & black pepper - .5 tsp. each
- Dried oregano - .5 tsp.
- Egg - 1
- Crumbled feta cheese - .33 cup
- Also Needed: 9x13-inch baking dish

Preparation Instructions:

1. Thaw and squeeze the water out of the spinach. Core and slice the bell peppers into halves lengthwise. Chop the tomatoes. Grate the zucchini and mince the white onion.
2. Warm up the oven to reach 350° Fahrenheit.
3. Add all of the fixings except for the cheese, tomatoes, and pepper into a container and mix well.
4. Arrange the peppers in the baking dish (cut side up). Fill each of the halves with the prepared stuffing. Add the tomatoes and sprinkle with cheese.
5. Place a lid on the dish or cover with foil.
6. Bake for about half of an hour. Take the top off and bake until the top is browned (approx. 25 minutes).
7. Serve immediately.

Stuffed Sweet Potatoes

Serving Yields: 4
Nutritional Calorie Count: 142.5

Ingredients Needed:

- Small sweet potatoes - 4
- Cooked black beans - 15 oz.
- Corn - 1 cup
- Thinly sliced green onions - 3
- Chopped cilantro - .5 cup

Ingredients Needed For The Vinaigrette:

- Lime - 2 - juice and zest
- Salt and ground black pepper - .5 tsp. each
- Honey - 2 tsp.
- Adobo sauce - 2 tsp.
- Olive oil - 1 tbsp.

Preparation Instructions:

1. Set the oven temperature to 350° Fahrenheit.
2. Whisk each of the fixings in a mixing container until well-combined.
3. Arrange the sweet potatoes on a baking sheet. Bake for 45 to 60 minutes.
4. Stir together the cilantro, onion, corn, and the beans.
5. Pour in the prepared vinaigrette, and toss until combined.
6. Once the potatoes are done, slice into halves lengthwise and let them cool for approximately 15 minutes.
7. Push down the center of each one to create a divot. You can use the back of a spoon. Add the prepared corn mixture and serve.

Dinner Specialties for Fall/Autumn

Braised Chicken & Artichoke Hearts

Serving Yields: 4
Nutritional Calorie Count: 707

Ingredients Needed:

- Olive oil - 1 tbsp.
- Chicken legs - 4 quarters
- Yellow onion - 1
- Garlic - 4 cloves
- Black pepper - 1 tbsp.
- Red pepper flakes - .5 tsp.
- Salt - 1 tsp.
- Chicken stock or low-sodium broth - 1-quart
- Canned artichoke hearts - 10
- Cherry peppers - 2 cups
- Lemons - juiced - 2
- Fresh thyme sprigs - 8
- Butter beans - 16 oz. can
- Also Needed: Dutch oven

Preparation Instructions:

1. Dice the onion and garlic. Drain the butter beans. Drain the artichokes and cut them in half.
2. Warm up the oven to reach 375° Fahrenheit.
3. Prepare the pan using the high heat setting and add the oil.
4. Sear the chicken until browned or about 5 minutes on each side. Set aside on a warm platter.
5. Stir in the garlic, onion, pepper flakes, salt, and black pepper. Cook for about 1 minute. Stir in the broth and let

it simmer for another minute or so. Remove from the heat.

6. Put the chicken back in the Dutch oven and add the thyme, lemon juice, cherry peppers, and artichoke hearts.
7. Put the pan in the oven to bake for about one hour.
8. Take the chicken out of the cooker and place in a warm platter again.
9. Stir the beans into the pan with the broth and artichoke mixture.
10. Place each leg quarter in a serving dish. Add a ladle of the artichoke, bean, and broth mixture over each serving.

Herb-Crusted Halibut

Serving Yields: 4
Nutritional Calorie Count: 273

Ingredients Needed:

- Panko bread crumbs - .75 cup
- Fresh parsley - .33 cup
- Fresh dill - .25 cup
- Fresh chives - .25 cup
- Extra-virgin olive oil - 1 tbsp.
- Finely grated lemon zest - 1 tsp.
- Sea salt - 1 tsp.
- Ground black pepper - .25 tsp.
- Halibut fillets - 4 - 6 oz.

Preparation Instructions:

1. Chop the fresh dill, chives, and parsley. Line a baking sheet with a layer of foil.
2. Warm up the oven to reach 400° Fahrenheit.
3. Combine the salt, pepper, lemon zest, olive oil, chives, dill, parsley, and the breadcrumbs in a mixing bowl.
4. Rinse the halibut well. Use paper towels to dry before baking.
5. Arrange the fish on the baking sheet. Spoon the crumbs over the fish and press into each of the fillets.
6. Bake until the fish is easily flaked and the top is browned or about 10 to 15 minutes.

Marinated Tuna Steak

Serving Yields: 4
Nutritional Calorie Count: 200

Ingredients Needed:

- Olive oil - 2 tbsp.
- Orange juice - .25 cup
- Soy sauce - .25 cup
- Lemon juice - 1 tbsp.
- Fresh parsley - 2 tbsp.
- Garlic clove - 1
- Ground black pepper - .5 tsp.
- Fresh oregano - .5 tsp.
- Tuna steaks - 4 - 4 oz. steaks

Preparation Instructions:

1. Mince the garlic, and chop the oregano and parsley.
2. In a glass container, mix the pepper, oregano, garlic, parsley, lemon juice, soy sauce, olive oil, and orange juice.
3. Warm up the grill using the high heat setting. Grease the grate with oil.
4. Add to tuna steaks and cook for 5 to 6 minutes. Turn and baste with the marinated sauce.
5. Cook another 5 minutes or until it's the way you like it. Discard the remaining marinade.

Pan Seared Salmon

Serving Yields: 4
Nutritional Calorie Count: 371

Ingredients Needed:

- Salmon fillets - 4 - 6 oz. each
- Olive oil - 2 tbsp.
- Capers - 2 tbsp.
- Salt and Pepper - .125 tsp. each
- Lemon - 4 slices

Preparation Instructions:

1. Warm up a heavy skillet for about 3 minutes using the medium heat setting.
2. Lightly spritz the salmon with olive oil. Arrange in the pan and increase the temperature setting to high.
3. Sear for approximately three minutes. Sprinkle with the salt, pepper, and capers.
4. Flip the salmon over and continue cooking for 5 minutes or until browned the way you like it.
5. Garnish with lemon slices and serve.

Penne with Shrimp

Serving Yields: 8
Nutritional Calorie Count: 385

Ingredients Needed:

- Penne pasta - 16 oz. pkg.
- Salt - .25 tsp.
- Olive oil - 2 tbsp.
- Red onion - .25 cup
- Minced garlic - 1 tbsp.
- White wine - .25 cup
- Diced tomatoes - 2 - 14.5 oz. cans
- Shrimp - 1 lb.
- Grated parmesan cheese - 1 cup

Preparation Instructions:

1. Peel and devein the shrimp. Dice the red onion and garlic.
2. Add salt to a large pot of water. Place on the stovetop and set to boil. Add the pasta and cook for 9 to 10 minutes. Drain.
3. Empty the oil into a skillet. Warm up using the medium heat setting.
4. Stir in the garlic and onion. Sauté until tender and mix in the tomatoes and wine. Continue cooking about 10 minutes, stirring occasionally.
5. Fold in the shrimp and continue cooking for 5 minutes or until it's opaque.
6. Combine the pasta and shrimp together and top it off with the cheese to serve.

Slow Cooked Lemon Chicken

Serving Yields: 6
Nutritional Calorie Count: 336

Ingredients Needed:

- Bone-in chicken breast halves - 6 - 12 oz. each
- Dried oregano -1 tsp.
- Seasoned salt - .5 tsp.
- Pepper - .25 tsp.
- Butter - 2 tbsp.
- Water - .25 cup
- Fresh parsley - 2 tsp.
- Minced garlic - 2 cloves
- Lemon juice - 3 tbsp.
- Chicken bouillon granules - 1 tsp.
- Optional: Cooked hot rice
- Also Needed: 5-quart slow cooker & skillet

Preparation Instructions:

1. Remove the skin from chicken. Pat it dry with paper towels.
2. Combine the pepper, seasoned salt, and oregano; rub over the chicken.
3. Prepare a skillet using the medium heat setting, and add the butter.
4. Brown the chicken. Transfer into the cooker.
5. Pour the water over the chicken.
6. Secure the lid and set on the low setting for 5 to 6 hours.
7. Baste the chicken with the cooking juices. Add the minced parsley. Place the lid on the pot and cook for 15 to 30 minutes longer.
8. Serve with a portion of rice if desired.

Speedy Tilapia with Avocado & Red Onion

Serving Yields: 4
Nutritional Calorie Count: 200

Ingredients Needed:

- Extra-virgin olive oil - 1 tbsp.
- Sea salt .25 tsp.
- Fresh orange juice - 1 tbsp.
- Tilapia fillets - four 4 oz. . - more oblong than square
- Red onion - .25 cup
- Sliced avocado - 1
- Also Needed: 9-inch pie plate

Preparation Instructions:

1. Combine the salt, juice, and oil together. Add to the pie dish. Work with one fillet at a time. Place in the dish and turn to coat all sides.
2. Arrange the fillets in a wagon wheel shaped formation so that one of each of the fillets are in the center of the dish with the other end draped over the edge of the dish.
3. Place a tablespoon of the onion on top of each of the fillets and fold the end into the center. When done. you will have four folded fillets with the fold against the outer edge of the dish.
4. Cover the dish with plastic wrap. Leave one corner open to vent the steam.
   Place in the microwave on high for 3 minutes. It's done when the center can be easily flaked.
5. Top the fillets off with the avocado and serve.

Snacks for the Fall/Autumn

Honey Nut Granola

Serving Yields: 6
Nutritional Calorie Count: 337

Ingredients Needed:

- Regular rolled oats - 2.5 cups
- Coarsely chopped almonds - .33 cup
- Cinnamon - .5 tsp.
- Sea salt - .125 tsp.
- Chopped dried apricots - .5 cup
- Ground flaxseed - 2 tbsp.
- Honey - .25 cup
- Vanilla extract - 2 tsp.
- Extra-virgin olive oil - .25 cup

Preparation Instructions:

1. Warm up the oven to reach 325° Fahrenheit.
2. Place a layer of parchment paper onto a rimmed baking sheet.
3. In a large skillet, combine the cinnamon, salt, almonds, and the oats.
4. Use the medium-high temperature setting and toast for about 6 minutes, stirring often.
5. Stir the oil, honey, flaxseed, and the apricots. Cook in the microwave for one minute. You can also use a small saucepan over medium heat for about 3 minutes.
6. Add the vanilla into the honey mixture and pour the oats in the skillet.

7. Spread out on the pan. Bake for approximately 15 minutes.
8. Cool completely and break into small pieces. Store in the refrigerator for up to two weeks.

Honey Rosemary Almonds

Serving Yields: 6
Nutritional Calorie Count: 149

Ingredients Needed:

- Raw - whole - shelled almonds - 1 cup
- Minced fresh rosemary - 1 tbsp.
- Sea salt - .25 tsp.
- Honey - 1 tbsp.

Preparation Instructions:

1. Use the medium heat setting to warm a skillet. Toss in the rosemary, salt, and almonds.
2. Drizzle with the honey and continue cooking for 3 to 4 minutes.
3. Stir often until the almonds are well coated and starting to darken around the edges
4. Transfer to the countertop. Use a spatula to spread the almonds evenly onto a pan coated with a spritz of nonstick cooking oil spray.
5. Cool for 10 minutes and break the almonds apart right before serving.

Italian Vanilla Greek Yogurt Affogato

Serving Yields: 4
Nutritional Calorie Count: 270

Ingredients Needed:

- Vanilla Greek yogurt - 24 oz.
- Sugar - 2 tsp.
- Hot espresso - 4 Shots or 0.75 of a cup strong brewed coffee
- Chopped - unsalted pistachios - 4 tbsp.
- Dark chocolate chips or shavings - 4 tbsp.

Preparation Instructions:

1. Spoon the yogurt into four tall glasses.
2. Mix .5 teaspoon of sugar into each of the espresso shots.
3. Pour one shot of hot espresso or 1.5 oz. of coffee into each of the yogurt glasses.
4. Top each one off with the chocolate chips and pistachios before serving.

Kale Chips

Serving Yields: 4
Nutritional Calorie Count: 56

Ingredients Needed:

- Olive oil - 1 tbsp.
- Chili powder - .5 tsp.
- Fine sea salt - .25 tsp.
- Steamed kale - 2-inch pieces
- Also Needed: 2 baking sheets

Preparation Instructions:

1. Warm up the oven to reach 300° Fahrenheit.
2. Line each of the pans with parchment paper.
3. Rinse and dry the kale. Add to a bowl with the olive oil.
4. Spread the kale out on the baking sheets (single layered). Roast for 25 minutes.
5. Let them cool for 5 minutes before serving.

Spiced Sweet Roasted Red Pepper Hummus

Serving Yields: 8
Nutritional Calorie Count: 64

Ingredients Needed:

- Garbanzo beans - drained - 15 oz. can
- Lemon juice - 3 tbsp.
- Roasted red peppers - 1 - 4 oz. jar
- Tahini - 1.5 tbsp.
- Minced garlic - 1 clove
- Cayenne pepper - .5 tsp.
- Salt - .25 tsp.
- Ground cumin - .5 tsp.
- Chopped fresh parsley - 1 tbsp.

Preparation Instructions:

1. Prepare all of the fixings in a food processor or blender.
2. When fluffy and smooth; add to a serving dish for at least one hour. Return to the room temperature when it is time to serve.

Walnut & Date Smoothie

Serving Yields: 2
Nutritional Calorie Count: 385

Ingredients Needed:

- Pitted dates - 4
- Milk - .5 cup
- Plain Greek yogurt - 2 cups
- Walnuts - .5 cup
- Cinnamon - .5 tsp.
- Pure vanilla extract - .5 tsp.
- Ice cubes - 2-3

Preparation Instructions:

1. Combine all of the fixings together.
2. Pulse in the blender until smooth and creamy.
3. Serve in chilled glasses.

Chapter 8: Recipes for the Winter Months

Breakfast Favorites for Winter

Barley Porridge

Serving Yields: 4
Nutritional Calorie Count: 354

Ingredients Needed:

- Wheat berries - 1 cup
- Barley - 1 cup
- Unsweetened almond milk - 2 cups (+) more for serving
- Blueberries - .5 cup
- Pomegranate seeds - .5 cup
- Water - 2 cups
- Roasted and chopped hazelnuts - .5 cup
- Raw honey - .25 cup

Preparation Instructions:

1. Pour the almond milk, water, wheat berries, and barley into a saucepan using the medium-high heat setting.
2. Once boiling, reduce the heat to the low setting. Let it simmer for 25 minutes.
3. Stir often. When done, top each serving with the pomegranate seeds, a tablespoon of honey, the blueberries, and hazelnuts. Give it a splash of the almond milk. Serve.

Christmas Breakfast Sausage Casserole

Serving Yields: 8
Nutritional Calorie Count: 377

Ingredients Needed:

- Ground pork sausage - 1 lb.
- Mustard powder - 1 tsp.
- Salt - .5 tsp.
- Eggs - 4
- Milk - 2 cups
- White bread - 6 slices - toasted & cut into cubes
- Mild Cheddar cheese - shredded - 8 oz.
- Also Needed: 9 x 13-inch baking dish

Preparation Instructions:

1. Grease the baking pan.
2. Crumble the sausage into a skillet and prepare using the medium heat setting. Drain when done.
3. Whisk the eggs with the milk, salt, and mustard powder.
4. Stir in the cheese, bread cubes, and sausage.
5. Pour into the prepared baking dish and place a cover on top.
6. Chill for at least 8 hours or overnight for best results.
7. Warm up the oven to reach 350° Fahrenheit.
8. Bake for 45 to 60 minutes.
9. Remove the lid, and lower the temperature to 325° Fahrenheit. Bake for 30 minutes or until set.

Crustless Spinach Quiche

Serving Yields: 6
Nutritional Calorie Count: 309

Ingredients Needed:

- Vegetable oil - 1 tbsp.
- Chopped onion - 1
- Frozen chopped spinach - 1 (10 oz.) pkg.
- Eggs - 5
- Shredded Muenster cheese - 3 cups
- Salt - .25 tsp.
- Ground black pepper - .125 tsp.
- Also Needed: 9-inch pie pan

Preparation Instructions:

1. Thaw and drain the spinach.
2. Warm up the oven to reach 350° Fahrenheit. Lightly grease the baking pan with cooking oil spray.
3. Heat up a skillet using the med-high heat setting. Toss in the onions and sauté until softened. Fold in the spinach and cook until the moisture is absorbed.
4. Whisk the eggs with the salt, pepper, and cheese. Add the thawed spinach mixture. Stir well and scoop into the pan.
5. Bake about 30 minutes. Let cool for about 10 minutes before serving.

French Toast Delight

Serving Yields: 12
Nutritional Calorie Count: 123

Ingredients Needed:

- All-purpose flour - .25 cup
- Milk - 1 cup
- Salt - 1 pinch
- Eggs - 3
- Ground cinnamon - .5 tsp.
- Vanilla extract - 1 tsp.
- White sugar - 1 tbsp.
- Thick slices bread - 12

Preparation Instructions:

1. Measure the flour and add to a mixing bowl. Whisk in the sugar, milk, vanilla extract, cinnamon, eggs, and salt.
2. Warm up a frying pan or lightly oiled griddle using the medium heat setting.
3. Soak the bread in the mixture until fully saturated.
4. Prepare each side of the French toast until golden brown.
5. Serve hot.

Fruit Bulgur Breakfast Bowl

Serving Yields: 6
Nutritional Calorie Count: 301

Ingredients Needed:

- 2% milk - 2 cups
- Uncooked bulgur - 1.5 cups
- Water - 1 cup
- Cinnamon - .5 tsp.
- Frozen/fresh pitted dark sweet cherries - 2 cups
- Dried/fresh chopped figs - 8
- Chopped almonds - .5 cup

Preparation Instructions:

1. Combine the cinnamon, water, milk, and the bulgur.
2. Stir once and bring to a boil. Put a top on the pot and lower the heat to medium-low.
3. Simmer for ten minutes or until liquid is absorbed.
4. Extinguish the flame, but leave the pan on the stove and stir in the cherries (if frozen no need to thaw), almonds, and figs.
5. Stir well to thaw the cherries and hydrate the figs. Stir in the mint, and scoop into serving bowls.
6. If desired, serve with warm milk or serve it chilled.

Greek Yogurt Bowl With Peanut Butter & Bananas

Serving Yields: 4
Nutritional Calorie Count: 370

Ingredients Needed:

- Medium bananas - 2
- Flaxseed meal - .25 cup
- Nutmeg - 1 tsp.
- Vanilla flavored Greek yogurt - 4 cups
- Peanut butter - .25 cup

Preparation Instructions:

1. Prepare four serving bowls with the yogurt. Top it off banana slices.
2. Put the peanut butter in a heatproof dish in the microwave to melt for 30 to 40 seconds.
3. Drizzle 1 tbsp. of the melted peanut butter over the sliced bananas. Sprinkle with the nutmeg and flaxseed meal. Serve right away and enjoy.

Marinara Eggs with Parsley

Serving Yields: 6
Nutritional Calorie Count: 122

Ingredients Needed:

- Extra-virgin olive oil - 1 tbsp.
- Chopped medium onion - .5 of 1 or 1 cup
- Minced garlic - 2 cloves or 1 tsp.
- Diced tomatoes - undrained - no-salt-added - 2 - 14.5 oz. cans
- Large eggs - 6
- Chopped Italian fresh flat-leaf parsley - .5 cup
- Optional: Crusty Italian bread with grated parmesan or Romano cheese

Preparation Instructions:

1. Prepare a skillet using the med-high heat setting and pour in the oil.
2. Dice the onion and toss it into the pan to sauté for about 5 minutes. Stir occasionally and add the garlic; continue stirring for another minute.
3. Add tomatoes with the juices into the pan and let it cook until bubbling for 2 to 3 minutes.
4. Crack an egg into a coffee mug.
5. Once the tomatoes are boiling, lower the heat to medium.
6. Use the spoon to make 6 indentions in the tomato mixture.
7. Add the egg to one of the slots and continue until you've used all of the eggs.
8. Place a top on the pot. Cook for 6 to 7 minutes or until they are the way you like them.
9. Top with the parsley and serve with bread and grated cheese if desired.

Lunch Options for the Winter

Chicken & White Bean Soup

Serving Yields: 6
Nutritional Calorie Count: 248

Ingredients Needed:

- Cooked cannellini beans - 15 oz.
- Cooked shredded chicken - 4 cups
- Leeks- .25-inch rounds - 2
- Freshly chopped sage - 1 tbsp.
- Chicken broth - 28 oz.
- Olive oil - 2 tsp.
- Water - 2 cups

Preparation Instructions:

1. Add the oil to a large saucepan and warm it up using the medium-high heat setting.
2. Cook for 3 minutes after adding the leeks. Stir in the sage and continue cooking 30 more seconds.
3. Pour in the water and chicken broth. Turn the heat to high and let it boil. Cover the pan and add the chicken. Stir. Cook for 3 minutes and uncover the pan.
4. Ladle the soup into the bowls and serve.

Chicken Marrakesh

Serving Yields: 8
Nutritional Calorie Count: 290

Ingredients Needed:

- Skinless breast halves - 2 lb.
- Cooked chickpeas - 15 oz.
- Large carrots - 2
- Large sweet potatoes - 2
- Diced tomatoes - 14.5 oz.
- Minced garlic - 1 tsp.
- Medium white onion - 1
- Salt - 1 tsp.
- Turmeric - .5 tsp.
- Dried parsley - 1 tsp.
- Cinnamon - .25 tsp.
- Ground cumin - .5 tsp.
- Black pepper - .5 tsp.
- Suggested: 6-quart slow cooker

Preparation Instructions:

1. Lightly grease the slow cooker.
2. Slice the chicken into 2-inch pieces. Peel and dice the carrots, sweet potatoes, and white onions. Mince the garlic.
3. Stir or whisk the cumin, parsley, turmeric, black pepper, and salt together.
4. Add everything into the greased cooker.
5. Secure the lid on the cooker and set the timer for 4 to 5 hours. The chicken should be done throughout and the potatoes should be tender.
6. Serve immediately.

Cucumber Dill Greek Yogurt Salad

Serving Yields: 6
Nutritional Calorie Count: 49.6

Ingredients Needed:

- Large cucumbers - 4 sliced
- Dried dill - 1 tbsp.
- Garlic powder - .25 tsp.
- Salt - .5 tsp.
- Ground black pepper - .25 tsp.
- Sugar - .5 tsp.
- Apple cider vinegar - 1 tbsp.
- Greek yogurt - 4 tbsp.

Preparation Instructions:

1. Combine all of the fixings except for the cucumber in a mixing dish. Whisk until well combined.
2. Add the sliced cucumbers and toss well.
3. Chill the salad for about 10 minutes in the fridge before serving.

Dill Salmon Salad Wraps

Serving Yields: 6
Nutritional Calorie Count: 336

Ingredients Needed:

- Salmon fillet - 1 lb. cooked or 3 - 5-oz. cans
- Carrots - .5 cup - 1 carrot
- Celery - .5 cup - 1 stalk
- Fresh dill - 3 tbsp.
- Diced red onion - 3 tbsp.
- Capers - 2 tbsp.
- Extra-virgin olive oil - 1.5 tbsp.
- Aged balsamic vinegar - 1 tbsp.
- Freshly cracked black pepper - .5 tsp.
- Sea salt or kosher salt - .25 tsp.
- Whole wheat flatbread wraps or soft whole wheat tortillas - 4

Preparation Instructions:

1. Prep the veggies. Dice the carrots, celery, and red onion. Chop the fresh dill.
2. Combine the vinegar, pepper, salt, oil, capers, red onion, dill, celery, carrots, and salmon in a large mixing bowl. Mix well.
3. Divide the salmon salad into your chosen bread. Fold it up or wrap it, and serve.

Fried Rice With Spinach – Peppers & Artichokes

Serving Yields: 4
Nutritional Calorie Count: 244

Ingredients Needed:

- Cooked rice - 1.5 cups
- Frozen chopped spinach - 10 oz.
- Marinated artichoke hearts - 6 oz.
- Roasted red peppers - 4 oz.
- Minced garlic - .5 tsp.
- Crumbled feta cheese with herbs - .5 cup
- Olive oil - 2 tbsp.

Preparation Instructions:

1. Prepare the vegetables. Mince the garlic. Thaw and drain the frozen spinach. Drain and quarter the artichoke hearts. Drain and chop the roasted red peppers.
2. Use the medium temperature setting on the stovetop to warm up a skillet. Warm up the oil. Toss in the garlic to cook for 2 minutes.
3. Toss in the rice and continue cooking for about 2 minutes until well heated.
4. Fold in the spinach and continue cooking for 3 more minutes.
5. Add the red peppers and artichoke hearts. Simmer for 2 minutes.
6. Stir in the feta cheese and remove the pan from the burner.
7. Serve immediately.

Italian Tuna Sandwiches

Serving Yields: 4
Nutritional Calorie Count: 347

Ingredients Needed:

- Extra-virgin olive oil - 2 tbsp.
- Freshly squeezed lemon juice - 1 medium lemon - 3 tbsp.
- Minced garlic - 1 clove - .5 tsp.
- Freshly cracked black pepper - .5 tsp.
- Drained tuna - 2 - 5 oz. cans
- Sliced olives - black or green - 2.25 oz. or about .5 cup
- Celery (1 stalk) or freshly chopped fennel - .5 cup
- Whole grain crusty bread - 8 slices

Preparation Instructions:

1. Whisk the lemon juice, pepper, garlic, and oil.
2. Drain and fold in the tuna, fennel, and olives. Break the chunks of tuna apart with a fork and stir well to combine all of the fixings.
3. Divide over four slices of bread and put the tops on to serve. Let the sandwiches sit for at least five minutes so the filling can soak up the bread before serving.

Mediterranean Bean Salad

Serving Yields: 4
Nutritional Calorie Count: 329

Ingredients Needed:

- Drained garbanzo beans - 15.5 oz.
- Drained kidney beans - 15 oz.
- Lemon - 1 juiced and zested
- Chopped medium tomato - 1
- Salt - .5 tsp.
- Chopped red onion - .25 cup
- Chopped fresh parsley - .5 cup
- Rinsed and drained capers - 1 tsp.
- Extra-virgin olive oil - 3 tbsp.

Preparation Instructions:

1. Combine all the fixings in a large bowl.
2. Cover with plastic or a lid and place in the fridge for about 2 hours.
3. Stir occasionally before serving.

Dinner Specialties for the Winter

Beef Cacciatore

Serving Yields: 6
Nutritional Calorie Count: 510

Ingredients Needed:

- Steak of choice - 1 lb.
- Red bell peppers - 2 medium
- Orange bell pepper - 1 medium
- White onion - 1 medium
- Olive oil - .25 cup
- Tomato sauce - 1 cup
- Black pepper - .5 tsp.
- Salt - 1 tsp.

Preparation Instructions:

1. Slice the beef into thin slices. Chop the peppers and onions.
2. Prepare until pureed a large pot using the medium heat setting. When hot, add the oil and beef. Cook for 7 to 10 minutes.
3. Toss in the onion. Sauté for 1 additional minute or until it starts to soften.
4. Add the peppers and cook for two more minutes. Sprinkle with the salt and pepper. Pour in the tomato sauce.
5. Stir and remove from the heat.
6. Add to a food processor, but leave the meat in the pot. Pulse for 1 minute until pureed.
7. Add the sauce back into the pot and mix well. Simmer five minutes using medium heat or until heated well. Stir constantly.
8. Serve with cooked pasta.

Beef With Artichokes – Slow Cooker

Serving Yields: 6
Nutritional Calorie Count: 416

Ingredients Needed:

- Stewing beef - 2 lb.
- Artichoke hearts - 14 oz.
- Kalamata olives - .5 cup
- Diced tomatoes - 14.5 oz. can
- Minced garlic - 2 tsp.
- Beef broth - 32 fluid oz.
- Ground cumin -.5 tsp.
- Dried oregano - 1 tsp.
- Dried parsley - 1 tsp.
- Dried basil - 1 tsp.
- Bay leaf - 1
- Grapeseed oil - 1 tbsp.
- Tomato sauce - 15 oz.
- Also Needed: 6-quart slow cooker

Preparation Instructions:

1. Drain and chop the artichokes into halves. Dice the garlic. Remove the pit from the olives and chop.
2. Add oil to a large pot using the medium-high heat setting.
3. Once it's hot, add the beef, and cook for about 2 minutes on each side.
4. Transfer the beef into the cooker and add the rest of the fixings.
5. Secure the lid and set the timer for 7 hours using the low heat setting.

Mediterranean Pork Chops

Serving Yields: 4
Nutritional Calorie Count: 161

Ingredients Needed:

- Boneless pork loin chops - 4 - .5-inch cut
- Salt - .25 tsp.
- Dried rosemary - 1 tsp.
- Ground black pepper - .25 tsp.
- Minced garlic - 1.5 tsp.

Preparation Instructions:

1. Warm up the oven to 425° Fahrenheit.
2. Season the chops with the salt and pepper. Set to the side.
3. Whisk the rosemary and garlic together. Rub into the pork chops.
4. Prepare a roasting pan with a layer of aluminum foil. Arrange the chops in it. Place in the oven.
5. Lower the temperature to 350° Fahrenheit and roast for 25 minutes.
6. Serve right away.

Nicoise-Style Tuna Salad with Olives & White Beans

Serving Yields: 4
Nutritional Calorie Count: 548

Ingredients Needed:

- Green beans - .75 lb.
- Solid white albacore tuna - 12 oz. can
- Great Northern beans - 16 oz. can
- Sliced black olives - 2.25 oz.
- Thinly sliced medium red onion - .25 of 1
- Large hard-cooked eggs - 4
- Dried oregano - 1 tsp.
- Extra-virgin olive oil - 6 tbsp.
- Lemon juice - 3 tbsp.
- Ground black pepper and salt - to taste
- Finely grated lemon zest - .5 tsp.
- Water - .33 cup

Preparation Instructions:

1. Drain the can of tuna, Great Northern beans, and black olives. Trim and snap the green beans into halves. Thinly slice the red onion. Cook and peel the eggs until hard boiled.
2. Pour the water and salt into a skillet and add the beans.
3. Place a top on the pot and turn the heat to high. Bring to a boil.
4. Once the beans are cooking, set a timer for 5 minutes. Immediately, drain and add the beans to a cookie sheet with a raised edge on paper towels to cool.
5. Combine the onion, olives, white beans, and drained tuna. Mix together with the zest, lemon juice, oil, and oregano.
6. Pour the mixture over the salad and gently toss.

7. Adjust the seasonings to your liking. Portion the tuna-bean salad with the green beans and eggs to serve.

Slow Cooked Roasted Turkey Breast

Serving Yields: 8
Nutritional Calorie Count: 333

Ingredients Needed:

- Boneless turkey breast - trimmed - 4 lb.
- Chicken broth - divided - .5 cup
- Fresh lemon juice - 2 tbsp.
- Chopped onion - 2 cups
- Pitted kalamata olives - .5 cup
- Oil-packed sun-dried tomatoes - thinly sliced - .5 cup
- Greek seasoning - such as McCormick's - 1 tsp.
- Salt - .5 tsp.
- Black pepper - .25 tsp.
- All-purpose flour - 3 tbsp.

Preparation Instructions:

1. Arrange the turkey breast, salt, Greek seasoning, tomatoes, olives, onion, lemon juice, and 1/4 cup of the chicken broth into the slow cooker. Secure the lid set the timer for 7 hours on the low setting.
2. Combine the rest of the broth with the flour in a small mixing container. Whisk until smooth and stir into the slow cooker at the end of the 7-hour cooking time.
3. Cover and continue cooking on low for another 30 minutes before serving.

Spanish Moroccan Fish

Serving Yields: 12
Nutritional Calorie Count: 268

Ingredients Needed:

- Vegetable oil - 1 tbsp.
- Onion - 1
- Garlic - 1 clove
- Garbanzo beans - 1 can - 15 oz.
- Red bell peppers - 2
- Large carrot - 1
- Tomatoes - 3
- Olives - 4
- Fresh parsley - .25 cup
- Ground cumin - .25 cup
- Paprika - 3 tbsp.
- Chicken bouillon granules - 2 tbsp.
- Cayenne pepper - 1 tsp.
- Salt - to taste
- Tilapia fillets - 5 lb.

Preparation Instructions:

1. Finely chop the garlic, onion, tomatoes, olives, and parsley. Drain and rinse the garbanzo beans. Slice the carrots and bell peppers.
2. Warm up the oil in a skillet using the medium heat setting.
3. Stir in the onion and garlic. Sauté until softened or about 5 minutes.
4. Stir in the bell peppers, olives, tomatoes, carrots, and the beans.
5. Simmer for about 5 more minutes.
6. Sprinkle with the paprika, cumin, parsley, chicken bouillon, and the cayenne over the veggies.

7. Dust with the salt and stir the vegetables. Add fish. Pour in enough water to cover the fish.
8. Set the temperature to low. Cook until the fish are flaky or about 40 minutes.

Sweet Sausage Marsala

Serving Yields: 6
Nutritional Calorie Count: 509

Ingredients Needed:

- Italian sausage links - 1 lb.
- Medium red bell pepper - 1
- Medium green bell pepper - 1
- Tomatoes - 14.5 oz. can
- Peeled large onion - .5 of 1
- Minced garlic - .5 tsp.
- Dried oregano - .125 tsp.
- Black pepper - .125 tsp.
- Marsala wine - 1 tbsp.
- Water .33 cup
- Uncooked bow-tie pasta - 16 oz.

Preparation Instructions:

1. Slice the onion and green peppers. Dice the tomatoes or purchase them precut.
2. Prepare a large pan of boiling water - about half full. Add the pasta and simmer for about 8-10 minutes.
3. Meanwhile, add the sausage to a medium skillet and pour in the water. Set using the medium-high heat temperature. Put a top on the pot and simmer for 8 minutes.
4. When the pasta is done, drain into a colander and set to the side for now.
5. Drain the sausage and return to the skillet. Stir in the wine, garlic, onion, and peppers. Simmer about 5 minutes using the medium-high temperature setting or until done.

6. Empty in the tomatoes and sprinkle with the oregano and black pepper.
7. Add the pasta and continue stirring. Remove the pan from the heat and serve.

Snacks for the Winter

Banana Sour Cream Bread

Serving Yields: 32
Nutritional Calorie Count: 263

Ingredients Needed:

- White sugar - .25 cup
- Ground cinnamon - 1 tsp.
- Butter - .75
- White sugar - 3 cups
- Eggs - 3
- Very ripe bananas, mashed - 6
- Sour cream - 16 oz. container
- Vanilla extract - 2 tsp.
- Ground cinnamon - 2 tsp.
- Salt - .5 tsp.
- Baking soda - 3 tsp.
- All-purpose flour - 4.5 cups
- Chopped walnuts (optional) - 1 cup
- Also Needed: 4 - 7 x 3-inch loaf pans

Preparation Instructions:

1. Warm up the oven to reach 300°Fahrenheit. Grease the loaf pans.
2. Sift the sugar and one teaspoon of the cinnamon. Dust the pan with the mixture.
3. Cream the butter with the rest of the sugar. Mash the bananas with the eggs and combine with the cinnamon, vanilla, sour cream, salt, baking soda, and the flour. Toss in the nuts last.

4. Pour the mixture into the pans. Bake for 1 hour. Test for doneness with a toothpick in the center. It's done when it comes out clean.

Chia Greek Yogurt Pudding

Serving Yields: 4
Nutritional Calorie Count: 263

Ingredients Needed:

- Chia seeds - .66 cup
- Hulled hemp seeds - 2 tbsp.
- Ground flaxseeds - 2 tbsp.
- Unsweetened soy milk - 1 cup
- Cinnamon - 1 tsp.
- Honey - 1 tbsp.
- Vanilla extract - 1 tsp.
- Greek yogurt - 1 cup

Preparation Instructions:

1. Whisk the milk and yogurt together in a large mixing dish.
2. Stir in the vanilla, cinnamon, honey, flaxseed, and hemp seeds.
3. Lastly, add the chia seeds and stir just enough to mix.
4. Place it in a container and chill for at least 15 minutes.
5. Stir again and chill for another hour. Serve as desired.

Chocolate Avocado Pudding

Serving Yields: 4
Nutritional Calorie Count: 295.3

Ingredients Needed:

- Large chilled avocados - 2
- Unsweetened cocoa powder - .33 cup
- Maple syrup - .33 cup
- Unsweetened vanilla extract - 2 tsp.
- Chopped hazelnuts - 4 tbsp.
- Full-fat coconut milk - unsweetened - .5 cup

Preparation Instructions:

1. Cut the avocados in half and remove the seeds. Scoop out the flesh and transfer to the food processor.
2. Add the rest of the fixings except for the nuts. Blend for 1 to 2 minutes until creamy smooth.
3. Spoon into four serving dishes and top with the nuts to serve.

Italian Apple Olive Oil Cake

Serving Yields: 12
Nutritional Calorie Count: 294

Ingredients Needed:

- Gala apples - 2 large
- Orange juice - for soaking apples
- All-purpose flour - 3 cups
- Ground cinnamon - .5 tsp.
- Nutmeg - .5 tsp.
- Baking powder - 1 tsp.
- Baking soda - 1 tsp.
- Sugar - 1 cup
- Extra-virgin olive oil - 1 cup
- Large eggs - 2
- Gold raisins - .66 cup
- Confectioner's sugar - for dusting
- Also Needed: 9-inch baking pan

Preparation Instructions:

1. Peel and finely chop the apples. Drizzle the apples with just enough orange juice to prevent browning.
2. Soak the raisins in warm water for 15 minutes and drain well.
3. Sift the baking soda, baking powder, cinnamon, nutmeg, and flour. Set aside.
4. Pour the olive oil and sugar into the bowl of a stand mixer. Mix on the low setting for 2 minutes or until well combined.
5. Blend while running, break in the eggs one at a time, and continue mixing for 2 minutes. The mixture should increase in volume, it should be thick - not runny.
6. Combine all of the ingredients well. Begin by making a well in the center of the flour mixture and add in the olive

and sugar mixture.

7. Remove the apples of any excess of juice and drain the raisins that have been soaking. Add them together with the batter, mixing well.

8. Prepare the baking pan with parchment paper. Spoon the batter into the pan and level it with the back of a wooden spoon.

9. Bake for 45 minutes at a 350° Fahrenheit.

10. When ready, remove the cake from the parchment paper and transfer into a serving dish. Dust with the confectioner's sugar. Warm up dark honey to garnish the top.

Maple Vanilla Baked Pears

Serving Yields: 4
Nutritional Calorie Count: 103.9

Ingredients Needed:

- Pears - 4
- Maple syrup - .5 cup
- Cinnamon - .25 tsp.
- Unsweetened vanilla extract - 1 tsp.
- For the Topping: Greek yogurt

Preparation Instructions:

1. Warm up the oven to reach 375° Fahrenheit.
2. Slice each of the pears into halves. Cut off a small sliver on the underneath side so it will lay flat.
3. Remove the seeds from the core and place on a baking sheet with the face side up and sprinkle with the cinnamon.
4. Whisk the syrup and vanilla. Drizzle over the pears. Save 2 tablespoons for the garnishing.
5. Place in the oven and bake for 25 minutes or until softened.
6. When done, place in the serving dishes and drizzle with the rest of the maple syrup mixture.
7. Serve with a dollop of yogurt.

Mediterranean Flatbread

Serving Yields: 6
Nutritional Calorie Count: 450

Ingredients Needed:

- Olive oil - 1 tbsp.
- Cooked cannellini beans - .66 cup
- Marinated artichoke hearts - 4 oz.
- Baby spinach - 2 cups
- Sliced medium avocado - .5 of 1
- Freshly torn basil leaves - .25 cup
- Halved cherry tomatoes - .5 cup
- Small red onion - .25 sliced
- Sea salt - .25 tsp. or as needed
- Freshly cracked black pepper - .125 tsp.
- Almonds - .25 cup
- Water - 2 tbsp.
- Crumbled feta cheese - 2 oz.
- Pita bread - 3 pieces

Preparation Instructions:

1. Heat up the oven to reach 350° Fahrenheit.
2. Prepare the food processor and add the water, oil, beans, almonds, pepper, salt, basil, and spinach. Pulse for one minute until creamy.
3. Spread the pita bread out on a large baking sheet. Spread with the prepared bean pesto.
4. Top it off with the artichokes, tomatoes, onion, and the avocado. Sprinkle with cheese.
5. Place the bread into the oven and bake about 10 minutes until they're crispy.
6. When ready, slice each piece into 4 segments and serve.

Serving Yields: 24 cookies
Nutritional Calorie Count: 187

Ingredients Needed:

- Vanilla extract - 1 tbsp.
- Extra-virgin olive oil - 1 cup
- Golden brown sugar - .75 cup
- Granulated sugar - .75 cup
- Kosher salt - 1 tsp. (+) extra for garnish
- Large egg - 1
- All-purpose flour - 2 cups
- Baking soda - .5 tsp.
- Semi-sweet chocolate chips - 2 cups

Preparation Instructions:

1. Warm up the oven to 350° Fahrenheit. Prepare 2 cookie tins with a sheet of parchment paper. Set to the side.
2. Pour in the vanilla, granulated sugar, brown sugar, olive oil, and the one tsp. of salt into a mixing container. Blend until it's creamy.
3. Whisk and add the egg.
4. Work in the baking soda and flour. Mix well and fold in the chocolate chips.
5. Use about 2 tbsp. for each cookie. Arrange on the baking sheets leaving about two inches between each one. Lightly sprinkle each one with the kosher salt.
6. Place the baking tins in the oven until the cookies are golden brown along the edges or about ten minutes.
7. Cool on the baking sheet for about 5 minutes.

Chapter 9: Recipes for the Spring Months

Breakfast Favorites for the Spring

Artichoke Frittata

Serving Yields: 4
Nutritional Calorie Count: 199

Ingredients Needed:

- Large eggs - 8
- Grated Asiago cheese - .25 cup
- Freshly chopped basil - 1 tbsp.
- Fine sea salt - .25 tsp.
- Black pepper - .25 tsp.
- Freshly chopped oregano - 1 tbsp.
- Olive oil - 1 tsp.
- Water-packed artichoke hearts - 1 can
- Chopped tomato - 1
- Minced garlic - 1 tsp.

Preparation Instructions:

1. Quarter and drain the artichoke hearts. Mince the garlic and chop the tomatoes, oregano, and basil.
2. Heat up the oven using the broil function.
3. Whisk the salt, pepper, eggs, oregano, basil, and cheese.
4. Prepare an ovenproof skillet over the med-high heat setting and olive oil.
5. Sauté the garlic for 1 minute. Remove the garlic from the skillet and stir in the egg. Add the garlic back into the mixture and sprinkle with the artichoke hearts and tomato.

Cook without stirring for 8 minutes. The center should be set.

6. Place your skillet in the oven to broil for 1 minute. The top should be lightly browned. Serve warm.

Greek Egg Frittata

Serving Yields: 6
Nutritional Calorie Count:107

Ingredients Needed:

- Eggs - 6
- Milk - .5 cup
- Diced tomatoes - .5 cup
- Spanish olives - .25 cup
- Kalamata olives - .25 cup
- Chopped spinach - 1 cup
- Salt - 1 tsp.
- Crumbled feta - .25 cup
- Pepper - .5 tsp.
- Oregano - 1 tsp.
- Also Needed: Quiche pan or 8-inch pie pan

Preparation Instructions:

1. Program the oven to 400°F. Grease the baking pan.
2. Whisk the milk and eggs. Add the remainder of the fixings. Stir well.
3. Bake until the eggs are set, usually about 15-20 minutes.

Greek Yogurt Breakfast Parfait with Roasted Grapes

Serving Yields: 4
Nutritional Calorie Count: 300

Ingredients Needed:

- Seedless grapes - 1.5 lbs. - 4 cups
- Extra virgin olive oil - 1 tbsp.
- 2% plain Greek yogurt - 2 cups
- Honey - 4 tsp.
- Chopped walnuts - .5 cup

Preparation Instructions:

1. Warm up the oven to reach 450° Fahrenheit with the pan inside.
2. Wash the grapes and discard the stems. Wipe with a towel and put in a bowl. Spritz with oil and toss to coat.
3. Bake for 20 to 23 minutes. They will look slightly shriveled. Stir about halfway through the cooking process.
4. Take the pan from the oven. Cool for five minutes.
5. Meanwhile, assemble the parfaits by adding the yogurt to the glass.
6. Once the grapes are cooled, garnish the yogurt with a teaspoon of honey, 2 tbsp. of the walnuts, and a portion of the grapes.

Greek Yogurt Pancakes

Serving Yields: 6
Nutritional Calorie Count: 258

Ingredients Needed:

- Blueberries - .5 cup
- All-purpose flour - 1.25 cups
- Salt - .25 tsp.
- Baking powder - 2 tsp.
- Sugar - .25 cup
- Baking soda - 1 tsp.
- Unsalted melted butter - 3 tbsp.
- Eggs - 3
- Greek yogurt - 1.5 cups
- Milk - .5 cup

Preparation Instructions:

1. Rinse the blueberries and drain.
2. Sift the flour, baking soda, sugar, baking powder, and salt in a dish.
3. In another container, add the milk, yogurt, and butter. Whisk well.
4. Gradually the egg mixture into the dry fixings. Let the mixture rest for about 20 minutes.
5. At that time, prepare a large skillet using the medium heat setting.
6. Add butter into the skillet to melt.
7. Pour in the pancake batter, cooking for about 2 to 3 minutes or until bubbly. Flip it over and continue cooking for 3 minutes or until browned.
8. When ready, place on a serving dish and garnish with a spoonful of yogurt and berries. Serve.

Mediterranean Egg – Pepper & Mushroom Cup

Serving Yields: 12
Nutritional Calorie Count: 67

Ingredients Needed:

- Chopped mushrooms - 1.5 cups
- Chopped roasted bell peppers - 1.5 cups
- Garlic powder - .5 tsp.
- Salt - .125 tsp.
- Black pepper - .25 tsp.
- Eggs - 10
- Olive oil - 2 tbsp.
- Coconut milk - .66 cup
- Freshly torn basil leaves - as desired
- Crumbled goat cheese - 2.5 tbsp.

Preparation Instructions:

1. Warm up the oven to reach 350° Fahrenheit.
2. Prepare the cups of a 12-count muffin tray with a spritz of olive oil and set aside. You can also use paper liners if you choose.
3. Crack the eggs into a bowl along with the milk, black pepper, salt, and garlic powder. Whisk well.
4. Add the pepper and mushrooms until well mixed. Divide evenly into each of the cups.
5. Bake for 25 minutes or until the muffins are set and browned.
6. When ready, remove the tray and let it cool for about 10 minutes.
7. Top the muffins with basil and goat cheese to serve.

Overnight Blueberry French Toast

Serving Yields: 10
Nutritional Calorie Count: 485

Ingredients Needed:

- Day-old bread - 12 slices
- Cream cheese - 2 (8 oz.) pkg.
- Fresh blueberries - 1 cup
- Eggs - 1 dozen
- Milk - 2 cups
- Vanilla extract - 1 tsp.
- Maple syrup - .33 cup
- White sugar - 1 cup
- Cornstarch - 2 tbsp.
- Water - 1 cup
- Fresh blueberries - 1 cup
- Butter - 1 tbsp.
- Also Needed: 9 x 13-inch baking dish

Preparation Instructions:

1. Cut the bread and cream cheese into 1-inch cubes.
2. Lightly grease a baking pan. Put half of the bread cubes into the dish and top with a layer of cream cheese cubes. Sprinkle with 1 cup of the berries and top of the remainder of the bread cubes.
3. Whisk the milk with the eggs, syrup, and vanilla extract. Empty over the bread cubes and refrigerate overnight with a plastic cover or lid over the container.
4. Transfer the dish to the countertop approximately 30 minutes before baking time.
5. Warm up the oven to reach 350° Fahrenheit.
6. Place the lid on the dish and bake for 30 minutes. Remove

the lid and continue to bake for 25 to 30 more minutes or until the surface is lightly browned.

7. Combine the water, cornstarch, and sugar in a medium saucepan. Stir constantly for 3-4 minutes.

8. Fold in the rest of the blueberries and reduce the heat. Simmer for 10 minutes until the berries start to burst. Stir in the butter and pour over the baked French toast.

Roasted Asparagus Prosciutto & Egg

Serving Yields: 4
Nutritional Calorie Count: 199

Ingredients Needed:

- Fresh asparagus - 1 bunch
- Minced prosciutto - 2 oz.
- Salt - .125 tsp.
- Ground black pepper - .25 tsp.
- Lemon - .5 of 1 - zest and juice
- Apple cider vinegar - 1 tsp.
- Olive oil - 2 tbsp. - divided
- Eggs - 4

Preparation Instructions:

1. Warm up the oven to reach 425° Fahrenheit.
2. Place the asparagus in a baking tray with 1 tbsp. of oil and set aside.
3. Warm up a medium skillet using the medium-low heat setting. Add the remainder of the oil when hot and place into the pan. Simmer 3 to 4 minutes until browned. Spoon this over the asparagus.
4. Sprinkle with the black pepper to coat and place the baking tray in the oven to cook for 10 minutes.
5. Remove the tray from the oven and toss the asparagus. Place back in the oven and continue cooking for 5 more minutes.
6. Prepare a pan over high heat. Once it's boiling, lower the heat to medium, and pour in the salt and vinegar.
7. Crack an egg into a measuring cup and gently add into the boiling water. Simmer for 4-6 minutes until it's firm, and the egg yolk has thickened - but not hard. Place on a paper-lined plate using a slotted spoon.
8. Continue with the other three eggs until done.

9. Once the asparagus is roasted, spritz with lemon juice and divide on to the four plates.
10. Top it off with the poached eggs and a sprinkle of lemon zest and black pepper before serving.

Lunch Options for the Spring

Chicken & Veggie Wraps

Serving Yields: 4
Nutritional Calorie Count: 278

Ingredients Needed:

- Plain Greek yogurt - .25 cup
- Chopped chicken - cooked - 2 cups
- Red bell pepper - .5 of 1
- English cucumber - .5 of 1
- Shredded carrots .5 cup
- Scallion - 1
- Fresh thyme - .5 tsp.
- Fresh lemon juice - 1 tbsp.
- Multigrain tortillas - 4
- Sea salt & black pepper - .25 tsp. each

Preparation Instructions:

1. Dice the cucumber, scallion, and bell pepper. Chop the chicken. Shred the carrot.
2. Mix each of the fixings into a large bowl.
3. Spoon the mixture into each of the tortillas.
4. Fold and serve.

Chickpea Salad

Serving Yields: 4
Nutritional Calorie Count: 163

Ingredients Needed:

- Cooked chickpeas - 15 oz.
- Diced Roma tomato - 1
- Diced green medium bell pepper - .5 of 1
- Fresh parsley - 1 tbsp.
- Small white onion - 1
- Minced garlic - .5 tsp.
- Lemon - 1 juiced

Preparation Instructions:

1. Chop the tomato, green pepper, and onion. Mince the garlic.
2. Combine each of the fixings into a salad bowl and toss well.
3. Cover the salad to chill for at least 15 minutes in the fridge.
4. Serve when ready.

Escarole with Garlic

Serving Yields: 4
Nutritional Calorie Count: 66

Ingredients Needed:

- Escarole - 1 head
- Salt - 1 tsp.
- Red pepper flakes - .125 tsp.
- Garlic - 1.5 tsp.
- Olive oil - 1.5 tbsp.

Preparation Instructions:

1. Tear the escarole leaves.
2. Use the medium heat setting on the stovetop to prepare a skillet.
3. Once it's hot, add the oil and garlic. Sauté one to two minutes until lightly browned.
4. Stir in the leaves and pepper flakes in batches. Season each batch with salt and toss well.
5. Continue cooking for about 5 minutes until the leaves have wilted. Serve immediately to enjoy at its best.

Goat Cheese Salad

Serving Yields: 4
Nutritional Calorie Count: 322

Ingredients Needed:

- Garlic - 1 clove head
- Fine sea salt - .125 tsp.
- Black pepper - .125 tsp.
- Freshly chopped basil - 2 tsp.
- Goat cheese - room temperature - 4 oz.
- Whole wheat bread - 8 slices
- Freshly shredded spinach - 2 cups
- Roasted bell peppers - cut into half and into strips - 2
- Olive oil - as needed

Preparation Instructions:

1. Warm up the oven to reach 350° Fahrenheit.
2. Remove the top from the garlic head. Once they are exposed, drizzle with olive oil before placing on the baking sheet.
3. Roast the garlic for 20 to 25 minutes until soft and fragrant. Set aside and let them cool.
4. Combine the salt, pepper, basil, one teaspoon of garlic, and the goat cheese to make a soft mixture.
5. Toast the bread and lightly spread with the goat cheese mixture. Top each slice off with a quarter of the roasted peppers and a heap of spinach. Put it together and serve.

Greek Shrimp Farro Bowl

Serving Yields: 2
Nutritional Calorie Count: 428

Ingredients Needed:

- Shrimp - 16
- Uncooked farro - 4 oz.
- Medium shallot - 1
- Persian cucumber - 1 medium
- Roma tomato - 1
- Parsley leaves - 2 tbsp.
- Black pepper - 1 tsp.
- Salt - 2.25 tsp.
- Oregano leaves - 1 tsp.

Preparation Instructions:

1. Do the prep. Peel and devein the shrimp. Slice the cucumber and dice the tomato. Peel and quarter the shallot. Chop the oregano leaves. Juice the lemon.
2. Add water to a small saucepan and use the high heat setting. Add .75 tsp. of the salt and bring to a boil.
3. Pour in the farro and cook for 15 minutes with a lid on the pan.
4. In a bowl, and the cucumber, tomato, shallots, mint, oil, cheese, and vinegar with .5 tsp. of the salt and .5 tsp. of the pepper. Toss well and set aside.
5. Drain the farro and set to the side for now.
6. Whisk .5 tsp. of the black pepper, one teaspoon of salt, and lemon juice in a large mixing bowl. Add the shrimp and oregano; toss well.
7. Warm up a large skillet using the medium-high heat setting. Pour in the oil. When hot, add the shrimp in a single layer and prepare for 2 minutes per side.
8. Divide the farro between two serving dishes and add the

cucumber salad topped off with shrimp.

9. Serve immediately and enjoy.

Mediterranean Tuna Salad

Serving Yields: 4
Nutritional Calorie Count: 328

Ingredients Needed:

- Cooked tuna in chunks - 12 oz.
- Small potatoes - 1 lb.
- Pimento stuffed green olives - .5 cup
- Sugar - 1 tsp.
- Green beans -1 lb.
- Ground black pepper - .5 tsp.
- Lemon juice - 1 tbsp.
- Brown mustard - 1 tbsp.
- Olive oil - 3 tbsp.
- For Serving: Chopped parsley & lemon wedges

Preparation Instructions:

1. Place a pot of water on the stovetop using the medium-high heat setting.
2. Add the potatoes. When boiling, reduce the heat setting and simmer for 5 minutes with the top on the pot until the potatoes are tender.
3. In a blender, pour in the lemon juice, mustard, pepper, olives, and sugar.
4. Mix until smooth or about 1 to 2 minutes.
5. Drain potatoes and veins. Divide the mixture into four serving platters.
6. Top it off with the olive mixture, and serve with lemon wedges.

Pasta With Sausage & Escarole

Serving Yields: 4
Nutritional Calorie Count: 333

Ingredients Needed:

- Uncooked bow-tie pasta - 3 cups
- Crumbled turkey sausage - 8 oz.
- Chopped escarole - 8 cups
- Diced fire-roasted tomatoes - canned - 14.5 oz.
- Small white onion - 1
- Red pepper flakes - 1 tsp.
- Minced garlic - 2 tsp.
- Salt - .25 tsp.
- Chicken broth - .75 cup
- Grated parmesan cheese - .25 cup
- Olive oil - 1 tsp.

Preparation Instructions:

1. Mince the garlic. Peel and chop the white onion and crumble the sausage.
2. Prepare a large saucepan with water and a little bit of salt.
3. Add the pasta once the water is boiling. Cook for 8-10 minutes.
4. Place a skillet on the stove over the med-high heat. Pour in the oil. When hot, add the onion and sausage. Sauté for about 5 minutes.
5. Add the broth, garlic, and escarole. Simmer for five more minutes until the escarole is tender.
6. Shake in the red pepper flakes and tomatoes. Simmer one more minute and remove the pan from the burner.
7. Drain the pasta into a colander. Add the escrow and toss until coated well.
8. Sprinkle with cheese and serve.

Dinner Specialties for the Spring

Chicken Thighs with Artichokes & Sun-Dried Tomatoes

Serving Yields: 6
Nutritional Calorie Count: 169

Ingredients Needed:

- Boneless chicken thighs - 6
- Julienne cut sun-dried tomatoes - 4 oz.
- Salt - 1.5 tsp.
- Grilled artichoke hearts - 14.75 oz. can
- Artichoke hearts liquid - .33 cup
- Minced garlic - 2 tsp.
- Black pepper - .75 tsp.
- Fresh parsley - 3 tbsp.
- Dried oregano - .5 tbsp.
- Suggested: 6-quart slow cooker

Preparation Instructions:

1. Drain the artichoke hearts (reserving .33 cup) and dice the sun-dried tomatoes. Mince the garlic cloves.
2. Sprinkle the chicken with the oregano, salt, and pepper. Arrange in a single layer in the cooker.
3. Add artichoke hearts, tomatoes, and garlic. Pour in the extra 1/3 cup of artichoke liquid.
4. Secure the lid and set the timer for 6 hours using the high heat setting.
5. When ready to serve, garnish with parsley.

Greek Honey & Lemon Pork Chops

Serving Yields: 4
Nutritional Calorie Count: 257

Ingredients Needed:

- Pork rib chops - 4
- Salt - .5 tsp.
- Cayenne pepper - .25 tsp.
- Lemon juice - 2 tbsp.
- Freshly snipped mint - 1 tbsp.
- Honey - 2 tbsp.
- Shredded lemon peel - 2 tbsp.
- Olive oil - 1 tbsp.

Preparation Instructions:

1. Remove all fat from the pork chops. Snip fresh mint and shred the lemon peel.
2. Slice the chops into 1-inch thick chunks, and put into a large resealable plastic bag.
3. Whisk the rest of the fixings and pour over the pork. Seal the bag.
4. Rotate the bag a few times and let it marinate for about 4 hours.
5. When ready to cook, prepare the grill. Grease the grilling rack with oil. Preheat using the medium heat setting.
6. Arrange the chops on the grilling rack. Grill for 5 - 6 minutes on each side. The meat thermometer should reach 160° Fahrenheit.
7. Serve immediately.

Greek Salad Tacos

Serving Yields: 4
Nutritional Calorie Count: 466

Ingredients Needed:

- Grilled chicken - 2 cups
- Black olives - .5 cup
- Romaine lettuce - 4 cups
- Tomatoes - 1 cup
- Cucumbers - .75 cup
- Cilantro - .25 cup
- Feta cheese - 1 cup
- Greek dressing - .5 cup
- Cucumber & Dill Dip - 1 cup
- Flour tortillas - 8

Preparation Instructions:

1. Do the preparation. Grill the chicken to your liking. Shred the lettuce and slice the black olives. Dice the tomatoes, cucumbers, and cilantro. Crumble the feta cheese and set aside.
2. Combine all of the fixings except for the tortilla, dip, dressing, and cheese.
3. Warm up the tortilla. Fill with the salad. Garnish with the dip and feta cheese.
4. Serve right way.

Grilled Lamb Chops with Mint

Serving Yields: 6
Nutritional Calorie Count: 238

Ingredients Needed:

- Lamb chops - 2.33 lb.
- Sea salt - 1 tsp.
- Red pepper flakes - .25 tsp.
- Minced garlic - 1 tsp.
- Freshly chopped mint leaves -.5 cup olive (+) more to garnish
- Olive oil - .33 cup

Preparation Instructions:

1. Prepare the grill with a generous amount of oil. Preheat using the medium-high heat setting.
2. Whisk the olive oil with the mint, pepper flakes, and salt. Use the rub over the chops.
3. Brush the chops with the mint oil and place on the grilling rack.
4. Cook for 3 to 4 minutes per side and put on the platter to serve.
5. Brush the chops with the remainder of the mint oil and a sprinkle of the mint. Serve.

Grilled Salmon

Serving Yields: 4
Nutritional Calorie Count: 214

Ingredients Needed:

- Salmon fillets - approx. - 4 - 5 oz. each
- Green olives - 4
- Minced garlic - 1 tbsp.
- Black pepper - .5 tsp.
- Fresh parsley - 1 tbsp.
- Fresh basil - 4 tbsp.
- Lemon - 4 slices
- Olive oil - as needed
- Lemon juice - 2 tbsp.

Preparation Instructions:

1. Chop the green olives, basil, and parsley. Thinly slice the lemon.
2. Warm up with the broiler. Use the high heat setting and place the cooking rack approximately four inches away from the heat source.
3. Whisk the lemon juice, parsley, basil, and garlic.
4. Lightly brush the fish with the oil mixture and sprinkle with the black pepper. Top it off with the prepared garlic mixture and place under the broiler.
5. Broil for 3 to 4 minutes. Place the fillets on aluminum foil. Continue to cook using the medium-low heat setting for approximately four minutes. When done, the fish will be opaque. The thickest part on a meat thermometer should read 145° Fahrenheit.
6. Transfer the salmon to a plate to serve with lemon slices and olives.

Mussels With Olives & Potatoes

Serving Yields: 4
Nutritional Calorie Count: 345

Ingredients Needed:

- Scrubbed mussels - 2.25 lb.
- Large peeled potatoes - 2
- Diced tomatoes - 14.5 oz.
- Sliced white onion - 1 medium
- Pitted green olives - .66 cup
- Minced garlic - 2 tsp.
- Cayenne pepper - .125 tsp.
- Salt - 1.5 tsp.
- Paprika - .5 tsp.
- Chopped fresh parsley - .5 cup
- Allspice - .125 tsp.
- Olive oil - 2 tbsp.
- Water - 1 cup

Preparation Instructions:

1. Peel the potatoes and cut into 1-inch cubes. Add to a pot of water, covering the potatoes with ¼-inch of water. Cover with plastic wrap.
2. Place in the microwave for 6 minutes using the high heat setting.
3. Prepare a large pot using the medium-high heat setting. Pour in the oil. When hot, toss in the garlic and onion. Simmer for 6 minutes.
4. Drain the potatoes and add to the cooker. Sprinkle with the allspice, paprika, pepper, and salt.
5. Stir well and simmer for 2 to 3 minutes. Pour in the tomatoes and water. Stir to remove the delicious brown bits from the bottom of the cooker.

6. Lastly, add the parsley, olives, and mussels. Simmer for 5 more minutes with a lid on. Serve immediately.

Salmon With Warm Tomato – Olive Salad

Serving Yields: 4
Nutritional Calorie Count: 433

Ingredients Needed:

- Salmon fillets - 4 - approx. 4 oz. - 1.25-inches thick
- Celery - 1 cup
- Medium tomatoes - 2
- Fresh mint - .25 cup
- Kalamata olives - .5 cup
- Garlic - .5 tsp.
- Salt - 1 tsp.
- Honey - 1 tbsp.
- Red pepper flakes - .25 tsp.
- Olive oil - 5 tbsp. (+) More for brushing
- Apple cider vinegar - 1 tbsp. (+) 1 tsp.

Preparation Instructions:

1. Slice the tomatoes and celery into 1-inch pieces and mince the garlic. Chop the mint and the olives.
2. Warm up the oven using the broiler setting.
3. Whisk 2 tbsp. of the olive oil, 1 tsp. of vinegar, honey, red pepper flakes, and 1 tsp. of the salt. Brush onto the salmon.
4. Line the broiler pan with aluminum foil. Spritz the pan lightly with olive oil, and add the fillets with the skin side down.
5. Place in the oven to broil for 4 to 6 minutes until well done.
6. Meanwhile, make the tomato salad. Mix .5 teaspoon of the salt with the garlic.
7. Prepare a small saucepan on the stovetop using the medium-high heat setting. Pour in the rest of the oil and add the garlic mixture with the olives and one tablespoon of

vinegar. Simmer for 3 minutes.

8. Prepare the serving dishes. Pour the bubbly mixture into the bowl. Add the mint, tomato, and celery. Dust with the rest of the salt and toss well.

9. When the salmon is done, serve with tomato salad.

Snacks for the Spring

Almond-Stuffed Dates

Serving Yields: 1
Nutritional Calorie Count: 149

Ingredients Needed:

- Whole almonds - 2 salted
- Pitted Medjool dates - 2
- Orange zest - .25 tsp.

Preparation Instructions:

1. Stuff each one of the dates with one of the almonds.
2. Prepare the zest and roll each of the prepared dates through the mixture.
3. Enjoy as a snack, anytime.

Date Wraps

Serving Yields: 16
Nutritional Calorie Count: 35

Ingredients Needed:

- Whole pitted dates - 16
- Thinly sliced prosciutto - 16 portions
- Black pepper - to taste

Preparation Instructions:

1. Wrap one of the prosciutto slices around each of the dates.
2. When done, serve with a shake of freshly cracked black pepper.

Mango Mousse

Serving Yields: 4
Nutritional Calorie Count: 358

Ingredients Needed:

- Medium ripe mangoes - 3
- Agave syrup - 3 tbsp.
- Coconut cream - 1.5 cup

Preparation Instructions:

1. Slice the mango to remove the stone.
2. Dice the flesh and place into a bowl. Mash them until smooth and puffy.
3. Add the coconut cream and whisk well. Whisk in the syrup. Spoon into the serving bowls.
4. Top off with a few chopped fruits and serve immediately.

Pistachio No-Bake Snack Bars

Serving Yields: 8 bars
Nutritional Calorie Count: 220

Ingredients Needed:

- Pitted dates - 20
- No-shell roasted & salted pistachios - 1.25 cups
- Rolled old fashioned oats - 1 cup
- Pistachio butter - 2 tbsp.
- Unsweetened applesauce - .25 cup
- Vanilla extract - 1 tsp.
- Also Needed: 8x8 baking dish

Preparation Instructions:

1. Use a food processor fitted with a metal blade.
2. Add the dates and process 30-45 seconds until pureed. Toss in the oats and pistachios. Pulse in 15-second intervals 2-3 times until a crumbly, coarse consistency achieved.
3. Place the applesauce, pistachio butter, and vanilla extract into the processor and pulse 20-30 seconds until dough is slightly sticky.
4. Line the pan with parchment paper.
5. Use a spatula to transfer the dough from the processor and pour into the pan. Press down firmly to evenly distribute the dough into the pan with another piece of parchment paper.
6. Lift the paper up and place evenly with the remaining 1/4 cup of no-shell pistachios onto the top of the dough.
7. Place the pan in the freezer with parchment paper on top and freeze for at least 1 hour before cutting.
8. Slice into 8 bars and store in an airtight container in the refrigerator for up to a week.

9. Note: To make pistachio butter, take 1 cup 'no-shell' pistachios and place in a food processor with 1 teaspoon vanilla extract. Process for 3-4 minutes, scraping down the sides as needed, until smooth.

Roasted Peaches & Blueberries

Serving Yields: 4
Nutritional Calorie Count: 45.7

Ingredients Needed:

- Peaches - 4
- Fresh blueberries - 1.5 cups
- Cinnamon - .33 tsp.
- Brown sugar - 3 tbsp.

Preparation Instructions:

1. Warm up the oven to reach 350° Fahrenheit.
2. Peel and slice the peaches. Arrange in a baking dish with the berries, a sprinkle of the cinnamon, and the sugar.
3. Use the broil setting. Let it cook for about 5 minutes and serve, or chill and serve.

Sautéed Apricots

Serving Yields: 4
Nutritional Calorie Count: 207

Ingredients Needed:

- Olive oil - 2 tbsp.
- Blanched almonds - 1 cup
- Sea salt - .5 tsp.
- Cinnamon - .125 tsp.
- Red pepper flakes - .125 tsp.
- Dried - chopped apricots - .5 cup

Preparation Instructions:

1. Prepare a frying pan using the high heat setting. Pour in the olive oil, almonds, and salt.
2. Sauté the almonds until golden which should take about 5 to 10 minutes. Stir frequently.
3. Spoon the almonds into a serving dish and add the chopped apricot, pepper flakes, and cinnamon.
4. Cool before serving.

Yogurt & Olive Oil Brownies

Serving Yields: 12
Nutritional Calorie Count: 150

Ingredients Needed:

- Olive oil - .25 cup
- Low-fat Greek yogurt - .25 cup
- Sugar - .75 cup
- Vanilla extract - 1 tsp.
- Eggs - 2
- Flour - .5 cup
- Cocoa powder - .33 cup (+) 1-2 tbsp. more if desired
- Baking powder - .25 tsp.
- Salt - .25 tsp.
- Chopped walnuts - .33 cup
- Also Needed: 9-inch square pan

Preparation Instructions:

1. Warm up the oven to 350° Fahrenheit.
2. Use a large spoon to combine the sugar, vanilla, and oil. Whisk the eggs and add to the mixture with the yogurt.
3. In another bowl, sift or whisk the flour, salt, cocoa powder, and baking powder. Stir in the olive oil mixture and the nuts and mix again.
4. Cover the pan with wax paper. Add the brownie mixture into the pan.
5. Bake for about 25 minutes. Let it cool thoroughly before removing the wax paper. Slice into squares.
6. Top it off with a portion of fresh berries of choice (add the extra calories.)

Conclusion

Staying busy is essential to combating food or drink cravings once you begin any new dieting technique. You need to remove the *craving* from your head, so you can break the hold it has on you. Try one or all of these suggestions. Organize your computer files. That could take a while if you are like most individuals.

Write in a journal about your health goals. Catch up on your favorite hobby or start one like drawing or painting to keep your hands and mind occupied. Look through some photo albums to break a smile. Call a friend and talk about anything that does not pertain to food or drinks. These are just a few of the things you can do to break the craving chain, but you get the idea.

Walk away with the knowledge learned and prepare a feast using your delicious new recipes and meal plan. Be the envy of the neighborhood when you provide a feast at the next neighborhood gathering. Show off your skills and be proud. You can also boast of how much better you feel using the Mediterranean diet plan.
Finally, if you found this book useful in any way, a review on Amazon is always appreciated!

Index for the Recipes

- Rosemary Thyme Lamb Chops
- Summertime Mixed Spice Burgers
- Tomato Feta Salad

Snacks For The Summer
- Chilled Dark Chocolate Fruit Kebabs
- Fruit - Veggie & Cheese Board
- Garlic Garbanzo Bean Spread
- Honey Lime Fruit Salad
- Strawberry Greek Frozen Yogurt
- Watermelon Cubes

Smoothies
- Mango Pear Smoothie
- Strawberry Rhubarb Smoothie

Chapter 7: Recipes for the Fall & Autumn

Breakfast Favorites For Fall/Autumn
- Avocado & Egg Breakfast Sandwich
- Baked Ricotta & Pears
- Feta & Quinoa Egg Muffins
- Ham & Egg Cups
- Mashed Chickpea - Feta & Avocado Toast
- Pumpkin Pancakes
- Scrambled Eggs With Goat Cheese & Roasted Peppers

Lunch Options For Fall/Autumn
- Avocado & Tuna Tapas

- Cannellini Bean Lettuce Wraps
- Greek Lentil Soup
- Mushroom Risotto
- Roasted Tomato Pita Pizzas
- Stuffed Bell Peppers
- Stuffed Sweet Potatoes

Dinner Specialties For Fall/Autumn

- Braised Chicken & Artichoke Hearts
- Herb-Crusted Halibut
- Marinated Tuna Steak
- Pan Seared Salmon
- Penne with Shrimp
- Slow Cooked Lemon Chicken
- Speedy Tilapia With Avocado & Red Onion

Snacks For The Fall/Autumn

- Honey Nut Granola
- Honey Rosemary Almonds
- Italian Vanilla Greek Yogurt Affogato
- Kale Chips
- Spiced Sweet Roasted Red Pepper Hummus
- Walnut & Date Smoothie

Chapter 8: Recipes For The Winter Months
Breakfast Favorites For Winter

- Barley Porridge

- Christmas Breakfast Sausage Casserole
- Crustless Spinach Quiche
- French Toast Delight
- Fruit Bulgur Breakfast Bowl
- Greek Yogurt Bowl With Peanut Butter & Bananas
- Marinara Eggs With Parsley

Lunch Options For The Winter

- Chicken & White Bean Soup
- Chicken Marrakesh
- Cucumber Dill Greek Yogurt Salad
- Dill Salmon Salad Wraps
- Fried Rice With Spinach - Peppers & Artichokes
- Italian Tuna Sandwiches
- Mediterranean Bean Salad

Dinner Specialties For The Winter

- Beef Cacciatore
- Beef With Artichokes - Slow Cooker
- Mediterranean Pork Chops
- Nicoise-Style Tuna Salad With Olives & White Beans
- Slow Cooked Roasted Turkey Breast
- Spanish Moroccan Fish
- Sweet Sausage Marsala

Snacks For The Winter:

- Banana Sour Cream Bread
- Chia Greek Yogurt Pudding
- Chocolate Avocado Pudding
- Italian Apple Olive Oil Cake
- Maple Vanilla Baked Pears
- Mediterranean Flatbread
- Olive Oil Chocolate Chip Cookies

Chapter 9: Recipes For Spring
Breakfast Favorites For the Spring

- Artichoke Frittata
- Greek Egg Frittata
- Greek Yogurt Breakfast Parfait with Roasted Grapes
- Greek Yogurt Pancakes
- Mediterranean Egg - Pepper - & Mushroom Cup
- Overnight Blueberry French Toast
- Roasted Asparagus Prosciutto & Egg

Lunch Options For The Spring

- Chicken & Veggie Wraps
- Chickpea Salad
- Escarole with Garlic
- Goat Cheese Salad
- Greek Shrimp Farro Bowl
- Mediterranean Tuna Salad
- Pasta With Sausage & Escarole

Dinner Specialties For The Spring

- Chicken Thighs With Artichokes & Sun-Dried Tomatoes
- Greek Honey & Lemon Pork Chops
- Greek Salad Tacos
- Grilled Lamb Chops With Mint
- Grilled Salmon
- Mussels With Olives & Potatoes
- Salmon With Warm Tomato-Olive Salad

Snacks For The Spring

- Almond-Stuffed Dates
- Date Wraps
- Mango Mousse
- Pistachio No-Bake Snack Bars
- Roasted Peaches & Blueberries
- Sautéed Apricots
- Yogurt & Olive Oil Brownies

Made in the USA
Lexington, KY
03 May 2019